FLEXIBLE SIGMOIDOSCOPY

FLEXIBLE SIGMOIDOSCOPY

Ronald M. Katon, M.D.

Professor of Medicine
Director, Gastrointestinal Diagnostic Unit

Emmet B. Keeffe, M.D.

Associate Professor of Medicine
Division of Gastroenterology

Clifford S. Melnyk, M.D.

Professor of Medicine
Head, Division of Gastroenterology

**Department of Medicine
Oregon Health Sciences University
Portland, Oregon**

Medical Illustrations by **Suzanne Moody**

Grune & Stratton, Inc.
(Harcourt Brace Jovanovich, Publishers)
Orlando   San Diego   New York
London   Toronto   Montreal   Sydney   Tokyo

Library of Congress Cataloging in Publication Data
Katon, Ronald M.
  Flexible sigmoidoscopy.

   Includes bibliographies and index.
   1. Sigmoidoscopy. I. Keeffe, Emmet B. II. Melnyk,
Clifford S. III. Title. [DNLM: 1. Sigmoidoscopy—
methods.   WI 620 K19f]
RC804.S47K38   1985   617'.5547   84-25116
ISBN 0-8089-1701-3

Grune & Stratton, Inc.
Orlando, FL 32887

Distributed in the United Kingdom by
Grune & Stratton, Ltd.
24/28 Oval Road, London NW 1

Library of Congress Catalog Number 7922-51
International Standard Book Number 0-8089-1701-3

Printed in the United States of America
85 86 87 88   10 9   8   7   6   5   4   3   2   1

To Ruth, Melenie, Melana, and our children
for their support and understanding.

Contents

Acknowledgments

We gratefully acknowledge support from the following companies in the preparation of this book.

    C-B Fleets, Inc., Lynchburg, Virginia

    Olympus Corporation, New Hyde Park, New York

    SmithKline Diagnostic, Inc., Sunnyvale, California

    Reichert Fiberoptics, Southbridge, Massachusetts

Foreword

I did my first sigmoidoscopy in 1948, but not until I read this remarkable book did I have a complete historical and practical perspective. This book tells you all you need to know about sigmoidoscopy.

Historians argue whether scientific knowledge advances because of the work of some great individual or simply because technological developments make uncovering new information easier. Derek Prince at Yale claimed that the discoveries Galileo made through his telescope were as much the result of the lens grinders' new-found abilities as of Galileo's unique perceptions. That is an argument beyond me, but clearly fiberoptic technology has put sigmoidoscopy literally within the grasp of all physicians, and has enlarged their diagnostic abilities.

When I visit a gastrointestinal service, I usually ask how many upper and lower endoscopies are done. Panendoscopy seems to be largely an exercise in caution and diagnostic pride, since there are safe and effective drugs to treat peptic ulcer and since we cannot do very much about gastric cancer anyway. I think that, even now, not enough sigmoidoscopies are carried out. After all, cancer of the colon remains (and has always been) the most common tumor of the gut, representing about 55% of all such cancers. I don't know whether small polyps turn into carcinomas as they grow or whether cancer is always cancer, but I do know that physicians can do something about cancer of the colon if they find it early enough, so fiberoptic sigmoidoscopy is very useful.

Despite the claim that the number of cancers in the right colon has increased over the past few decades, most cancers and polyps of the colon turn up in the sigmoid, which is, therefore, the segment of the colon that deserves the greatest scrutiny. Some enthusiasts claim that a total colonoscopy should be carried out in any patient who undergoes a fiberoptic sigmoidoscopy, to search out and destroy all polyps. Someday that may be possible, but because we do not yet have the legion of physicians and technicians trained to scrutinize every centimeter of the colon, a more practical approach is to examine the segment where most tumors are found.

Fiberoptic sigmoidoscopy is important for another reason. While a good radiologist can scrutinize the bowel with an air-contrast barium enema almost as well as a colonoscopist, a radiologist cannot perform a biopsy or remove polyps. Moreover, radiologists skilled in barium studies are fast disappearing. Most young radiologists-in-training prefer interventional forms of radiology and have little interest in looking at barium-filled guts. In many hospitals and private practice, radiologists defer more and more to sigmoidoscopists and colonoscopists.

This book, written by several skilled authorities, will give you an excellent introduction, almost a graduate course, in sigmoidoscopy. Although I wish that doctors did not always equate "to see" with "to know," for the rectosigmoid there is no better way to know what is going on than to see it through the fiberoptic sigmoidoscope. Read this book, practice with an expert, and you will see—and know—what you are doing.

Howard Spiro, M.D.
Professor of Medicine
Yale University School of Medicine

Preface

Over the past five years, flexible sigmoidoscopy has been the subject of a rapidly expanding literature and has captured the interest of diverse groups of physicians practicing primary care medicine. The instrument manufacturers have recognized this broad interest in flexible sigmoidoscopy and are competing for the market with a confusing array of instruments of variable lengths, capabilities, and costs. With this high level of physician interest and rapid proliferation of flexible sigmoidoscopes, a number of controversies have evolved. The merits of flexible versus rigid sigmoidoscopy, the optimal length of a flexible sigmoidoscope, and the question of adequate training and competence for nonspecialists in the field all remain unsettled. In this book we will address all of these topics and a number of other issues relevant to flexible sigmoidoscopy. Our primary goals in compiling this material are (1) to outline the indications and demonstrate the technique of flexible sigmoidoscopy; (2) to provide a practical guide to instrument design, purchase, and maintenance; (3) to organize and critique the published data regarding flexible sigmoidoscopy, and (4) to offer our opinions regarding the unresolved controversies in this area.

A young trainee who requests a "flex sig" on a patient may not realize that just a few years ago flexible sigmoidoscopy was not available. For over 100 years, rigid sigmoidoscopy was the time-honored method of examining the rectum and sigmoid colon. By the mid 1970s colonoscopy revolutionized the diagnosis and management of colonic diseases by gastroenterologists and colorectal surgeons, but sigmoidoscopy was still routinely performed with rigid instruments. In 1977 our group reported the superiority of 60-cm flexible sigmoidoscopy over standard rigid sigmoidoscopy, and several other studies later confirmed these findings. Rapid acceptance of flexible sigmoidoscopy, however, did not follow. Instead, a great deal of controversy developed over its proper application. Some experienced colonoscopists feared inappropriate substitution of flexible sigmoidoscopy for total colonoscopy. Others argued that 60-cm flexible sigmoidoscopy could not be readily mastered by nonendoscopists for widespread use in general practice. Shorter 35-cm flexible sigmoidoscopes were soon manufactured, but the availability of yet another instrument to visualize the distal colon and rectum generated further controversy. During this time, many gastroenterologists and colorectal surgeons substituted 60-cm flexible for rigid sigmoidoscopy in their routine practices. Time will tell which of the flexible sigmoidoscope lengths beomes most popular. It seems likely, however, that within the next several years flexible sigmoidoscopy with either a 60-cm or 35-cm instrument will largely replace rigid sigmoidoscopy.

With the recent rapid change in approach to sigmoidoscopy, we recognized the need for a comprehensive treatise on flexible sigmoidoscopy aimed primarily at the primary care practitioner. In this book we provide the novice endoscopist with a thorough description of the proper technique of flexible sigmoidoscopy. We also discuss other important topics in this area such as indications, contraindications, complications, a standard sigmoidoscopy medical record form, issues regarding screening for colorectal neoplasia, a consumer guide to the many available instruments, and basic information regarding the principles of fiberoptics and instrument care and maintenance. Finally, we share with the reader our interpretation of the controversies in this rapidly expanding area. Our hope is that this book will facilitate the introduction of flexible sigmoidoscopy to primary care providers and other new endoscopists, and will become a permanent resource of information regarding this important procedure.

The authors wish to express their gratitude to Pamela Briggs, Linda Clevinger, and Kathleen Alexander for their superb secretarial assistance. We are also very grateful to Monica Arntson and Jeanne DeBernardi, our faithful gastrointestinal assistants, for their many practical suggestions.

1

Historical Perspective: From Rigid to Flexible Sigmoidoscopy

The desire to visualize the rectum and distal colon has presented a challenge to physicians for many centuries. The earliest known treatise devoted completely to anorectal diseases is the *Chester Beatty Medical Papyrus* written by the Egyptians in the 12th to 13th century, B.C.[1] This papyrus is evidence for the antiquity of proctology. Hippocrates (460–377 B.C.)[2] mentions the use of a rectal speculum for the diagnosis and treatment of anal disorders. Later, John of Arderne from England (1307–1390)[3] was in demand for his treatment of anal disorders, which were a common occupational hazzard of knights in armor who spent long periods of time on horseback. These illustrations demonstrate a continued interest in proctology that spans many centuries.

HISTORY OF SIGMOIDOSCOPY

The need for internal examination of the rectum and colon has been recognized throughout history, but technological problems limited progress in this area. The following dates and events represent a brief sketch of important developments in colorectal endoscopy.

1809　Philipp Bozzini[21] of Germany is credited as the inventor of the first illuminating endoscope using a candle as a light source. His instrument was developed primarily for cystoscopic examination.

1853　Antonin Desormeaux[5] of France made a major improvement in endoscopic light sources by using a lamp that burned a mixture of alcohol and turpentine and reflecting this light source off a mirror. His endoscope is generally considered to have provided the first reasonable view of the rectum.

1865   Sir Francis Richard Cruise[21] of Ireland improved the quality of illumination by using a lamp that burned a mixture of petroleum and camphor.

1879   Max Nitze[21] of Germany made use of the newly invented electrical incandescent lamp as a light source for endoscopy. The application of electricity for sigmoidoscopic illumination was a considerable developmental milestone.

1895   Howard A. Kelly[21] of the United States is considered by some historians as the father of modern rigid proctosigmoidoscopy. He introduced straight metal tubes of different sizes and used the illumination technique of reflected light from a head mirror.

1899   J. R. Pennington[21] of the United States developed air insufflation via a rubber bulb and a cap that sealed the proximal opening of the sigmoidoscope. He also introduced distal illumination by engineering electric light transmission through an auxillary channel within the lumen of the endoscope.

1905   Herman Strauss[21] of Germany introduced a sigmoidoscope that had both distal rod illumination and air insufflation capabilities.

1912   Frank C. Yeomans[21] of the United States introduced proximal electrical illumination so that instruments could have both a proximal and distal light source.

1958   Hirschowitz et al.[10] reported their experience with the fiberoptic gastroscope and emphasized the flexibility and illumination capabilities of fiber optics. Hirschowitz's development is the first application of fiberoptic technology for examination of the gastrointestinal tract.

1959   Japanese workers[24] introduced the sigmoidcamera following successful development and use of the gastrocamera. This instrument provided pictures of the colonic mucosa to the level of the sigmoid colon but did not allow direct visualization.

1960   Japanese investigators[24] reported their experience in attempting to use the fiberoptic gastroscope for examination of the rectum and colon.

1963   R. Turell[20] of the United States reported the application of fiberoptics for sigmoidoscopic light transmission for both distal and proximal illumination in a rigid sigmoidoscope and highlighted its superiority over previous illumination sources. A flexible fiberoptic coloscope was discussed but no details regarding its clinical use were provided.

1965   Japanese endoscopists[26] described their initial attempt at fiberoptic colonic endoscopy and the difficulties of negotiating the sigmoid colon.

1968   Overholt[13] of the United States reported the first clinical experience with the fibersigmoidoscope. In 1969,[14] he demonstrated the utility of the fiberoptic flexible sigmoidoscope by successfully examining the colon beyond the 25-cm limit of rigid sigmoidoscopy. Visualization of the colon was impaired by the poor quality of these initial fiberoptic bundles and by the limited maneuverability of the sigmoidoscope secondary to inefficient distal tip manipulation. Niwa et al.[12] of Japan and Dean and Shearman[7] of England reported similar experiences.

1969   Provenzale and Revignas[16] of Italy used an end-to-end technique wherein the fiberoptic endoscope was guided into the large bowel by a polyvinyl tube positioned by prior transintestinal intubation.

1971   Overholt[15] described instrument improvements with wider angle vision and two-way tip deflection. Image transmission was improved by new fiberoptic bundles.

1971   Wolff and Shinya[24] of the United States and Salmon et al.[18] of England reported the superiority of the 86-cm fiberoptic colonoscope over rigid sigmoidoscopy. Wolff and Shinya later extended colon assessment to full colonoscopy utilizing the 186-cm colonofiberscope. They demonstrated the diagnostic and therapeutic utility of fiberoptic colonoscopy.[25] This experience represented a major advance in colonic surgery, since colonic polyps could now be removed via colonoscopic snare cautery without abdominal surgery. This report led to revolutionary changes in fiberoptic colonoscopy with emphasis on long colonoscopy and engineering improvements in instrumentation.

1977   Fiberoptic colonoscopy was in widespread use and of proven value, but sigmoidoscopy was still being performed with the rigid instrument. Bohlman et al.[4] at our medical center evaluated 60-cm fiberoptic flexible sigmoidoscopy in comparison with rigid sigmoidoscopy. The 60-cm instrument had four-way tip deflection and good optics. They demonstrated superiority of 60-cm sigmoidoscopy in terms of (1) less patient discomfort; (2) greater length of the colon examined; (3) 3–4 times greater yield of polyps and cancer; (4) minimal increase in performance time; and (5) convenience as an outpatient/office procedure. Controversy developed regarding whether a short instrument was needed and who was qualified to perform flexible sigmoidoscopy.

1979   Winawer et al.[22] of the United States studied 60-cm fiberoptic flexible sigmoidoscopy and verified the findings of Bohlman et al. They suggested that routine colorectal screening for polyps and cancer might be performed by nonendoscopists using a shorter 30-cm flexible instrument.

1982   Winawer et al.[23] trained a nonendoscopist primary care physician to use a 30-cm flexible sigmoidoscope and demonstrated that a short flexible instrument could be substituted for a rigid sigmoidoscope in an office setting.

1983   Grobe et al.[9] did a comparative study of 35-cm flexible sigmoidoscopy versus rigid sigmoidoscopy. The inexpensive flexible instument had only two-way tip deflection, manual suction, and bulb insufflation. Both the rigid and 35-cm flexible examination required four minutes to perform. However, the flexible instrument allowed a one-third greater insertion distance, less patient discomfort, and detected more than twice the number of polypoid lesions than the rigid sigmoidoscope.

1984   Zucker et al.[27] compared 30-cm flexible sigmoidoscopy to 60-cm flexible sigmoidoscopy in symptomatic patients. They found that sigmoidoscopy performed with the 60-cm compared to the 30-cm instrument was not associated with a significantly increased yield of colonic polypoid lesions. They demonstrated that the majority of neoplastic lesions were beyond the limit of rigid sigmoidoscopy but within the range of the 30-cm instrument.

1984   Dubow et al.[8] at our medical center performed a comparative study of short (35-cm) versus long (60-cm) flexible sigmoidoscopy in screening asymptomatic patients for colorectal neoplasia. They found that the 35-cm flexible sigmoidoscope (1) examined almost twice the distance of an average rigid sigmoidoscopy; (2) was more rapidly performed; (3) was better tolerated and preferred by patients; and (4) detected 76% of all polyps.

From a historical perspective, it seems ironic that by July 1969 the United States had the technological capability of putting a man on the moon, but was only in the early developmental stage of flexible sigmoidoscopy.

LIMITATIONS OF RIGID SIGMOIDOSCOPY

The major indications for sigmoidoscopy, which apply to both rigid and flexible sigmoidoscopy, are diagnosis of colorectal diseases, screening asymptomatic individuals for colonic neoplasia, surveillance of high-risk patient groups for cancer, and therapy such as snare polypectomy. However, major limitations of rigid sigmoidoscopy in achieving these goals have been recognized and noted in the literature. The length of bowel examined by rigid sigmoidoscopy is limited. Since mean insertion distance is 18–19 cm using rigid sigmoidoscopy,[11] examination is primarily an assessment of the rectum and distal sigmoid (Fig. 1-1). Underutilization also represents a problem.[17] Patient acceptance and physician application of rigid sigmoidoscopy has been poor. There is a general reluctance by physicians to use sigmoidoscopy for a routine screening examination of patients over 50 years of age or prior to x-ray studies of the colon. This poor compliance may be due to a number of factors including lack of public awareness of the importance of colorectal disease, limited training of physicians in sigmoidoscopy, high cost-benefit ratio in asymptomatic patients (i.e., a large number of patients must be screened to uncover a small number of neoplasms), and patient discomfort during examination. Recent studies point to a change in site distribution of colon cancers from the rectum to the sigmoid and more proximal colon.[19] A previous 65–70% incidence rate of colon cancer in the distal 25 cm of the rectosigmoid area has been reduced to approxi-

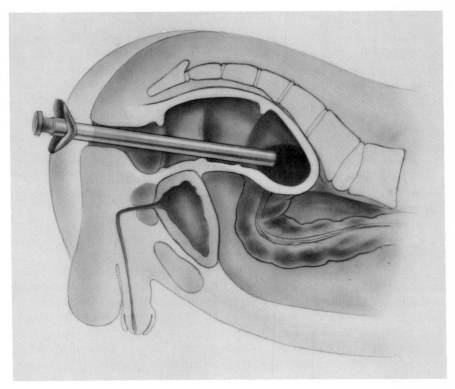

Figure 1-1. The insertion of the rigid sigmoidoscope to the rectosigmoid junction demonstrating its acute angulation.

mately 50–55%.[6] This is further compounded by (1) the practical limitation of rigid sigmoidoscopy insertion distance being 18–19 cm,[11] and (2) the findings in recent studies which demonstrate a 27% false-negative rate from examination by rigid sigmoidoscopy of the 16 cm to 25 cm area.[4,6] This implies that rigid sigmoidoscopy is most effective in the distal 16 cm of the rectosigmoid colon with a potential discovery rate of only 20–30% of colorectal cancers. Finally, rigid sigmoidoscopy has limited accuracy in certain types of colitis with rectal sparring, i.e., Crohn's disease, ischemic colitis, and antibiotic-associated colitis.

In spite of the limitations of rigid sigmoidoscopy noted, several reasonable indications for rigid sigmoidoscopy still exist. These include (1) examination of the rectal mucosa of patients too ill to undergo bowel preparation; (2) evaluation of mucosa in managing inflammatory bowel disease; (3) localization of rectal lesions prior to surgical removal; (4) and rectal submucosal biopsy for systemic disease such as amyloidosis. Directed deep biopsies are better obtained through the rigid instrument.

ADVANTAGES AND DISADVANTAGES OF FLEXIBLE SIGMOIDOSCOPY

Flexible sigmoidoscopy is a major advance in the diagnosis of colorectal disorders. The application of fiber optics and modern engineering has produced instruments capable of good flexibility, easy maneuverability, excellent illumination, full photographic capabilities, and therapeutic application. These qualities are being recognized by an increasing percentage of general physicians. With proper training and experience, the previous underutilization of sigmoidoscopy can probably be overcome. In addition, the flexible instrument has higher patient acceptance than rigid sigmoidoscopy. The colonic mucosal surface examined can be at least doubled and result in a greater diagnostic yield. Flexible sigmoidoscopy is superior to rigid sigmoidoscopy as a screening test for colorectal neoplasia.[4,9] There may be less reluctance to perform flexible sigmoidoscopy before ordering a barium enema as part of the evaluation in a patient with lower abdominal complaints. Future technological advances may further simplify use of these instruments.

The drawbacks of flexible sigmoidoscopy are increased cost, increased procedure time, and the requirement for some training. Costs are related to the initial purchase price of the basic equipment, consisting of instrument and light source, and also higher maintenance costs. Physician fees for 60-cm flexible sigmoidoscopy range from 2–3 times their usual fee for rigid sigmoidoscopy. Manufacturers have responded to these criticisms by offering less expensive instruments. The 60-cm instrument has been extremely durable and has practically replaced the rigid sigmoidoscope in our diagnostic unit. Further studies are needed to determine the utility and maintenance costs of the shorter flexible instrument.

The increased time required to perform flexible sigmoidoscopy is related to both performance time and time required to clean the equipment. Flexible sigmoidoscopy with the 60-cm instrument generally requires twice the time of rigid sigmoidoscopy (10 min versus 5–6 min).[4] However, this time period lengthens when additional studies or photography are performed. Equipment disinfection and cleaning requires 10–12 minutes for completion, resulting in a total time commitment of approximately 20 minutes per procedure.

There has been considerable controversy regarding the requirements for "certification" to perform flexible sigmoidoscopy using the 60-cm instrument. There have been concerns over the risk of increased complications related to negotiation of the sigmoid curves.

The advent of the 35-cm flexible sigmoidoscope eliminates some of this concern and allows for more direct comparison of rigid versus flexible sigmoidoscopy. A study with 35-cm flexible sigmoidoscopy compared to rigid sigmoidoscopy has shown favorable results for the 35-cm examination with equal time required to perform the procedure, greater area examined, increased yield of pathology, and greater patient comfort.[9] Since this shorter instrument does not traverse the entire sigmoid colon, expertise in its use should be easily acquired. Flexible sigmoidoscopy may in the near future be more widely utilized by primary care nonendoscopists as an office procedure in screening asymptomatic patients for colorectal neoplasia and evaluating lower abdominal symptoms.

REFERENCES

1. Banov L: The Chester Beatty Medical Papyrus: The earliest known treatise completely devoted to anorectal diseases. Surgery 58:1037–1043, 1965.
2. Banov L: Hippocratic proctology. Southern Med J 60:667–670, 1967.
3. Bettmann OL: A Pictorial History of Medicine: John of Arderne. Springfield, Charles C. Thomas, 1956, p 84.
4. Bohlman T, Katon RM, Lipshutz G, et al.: Fiberoptic pansigmoidoscopy—an evaluation and comparison with rigid sigmoidoscopy. Gastroenterology 72:644–649, 1977.
5. Brown CH: Proctosigmoidoscopy: General remarks, in Brown CH (Ed): Diagnostic Procedures in Gastroenterology. St. Louis, C.V. Mosby, 1967, p 213–225.
6. Crespi M, Weissman GS, Gilbertsen VA, et al.: The role of proctosigmoidoscopy in screening for colorectal neoplasia. CA 34:158–166, 1984.
7. Dean ACB, Shearman DJC: Clinical evaluation of a new fibreoptic colonoscope. Lancet 1:550–552, 1970.

8. Dubow RA, Katon RM, Benner KG, et al.: Short (35-cm) vs. long (60-cm) flexible sigmoidoscopy: A comparison of findings and tolerance in asymptomatic patients. Gastrointest Endosc (abstract) 30:142, 1984.

9. Grobe JL, Kozarek RA, Sanowski RA: Flexible versus rigid sigmoidiscopy: A comparison using an inexpensive 35-cm flexible proctosigmoidoscope. Am J Gastroenterol 78:569–571, 1983.

10. Hirschowitz BI, Curtiss LE, Peters CW, Pollard HM: Demonstration of a new gastroscope, the "Fiberscope." Gastroenterology 35:50–53, 1958.

11. Nivatvongs S, Fryd DS: How far does the proctosigmoidoscope reach? A prospective study of 1000 patients. N Engl J Med 303:380–382, 1980.

12. Niwa H, Utsumi Y, Kanebo E, et al: Clinical experience of colonic fiberscope. Jap J Gastroenterol 66:907–917, 1969.

13. Overholt BF: Clinical experience with the fibersigmoidoscope. Gastrointest Endosc 15:27, 1968.

14. Overholt BF: Flexible fiberoptic sigmoidoscopes. CA 19:81–84, 1969.

15. Overholt BF: Flexible fiberoptic sigmoidoscopy. Technique and preliminary results. Cancer 28:123–126, 1971.

16. Provenzale L, Revignas A: An original method for guided intubation of the colon. Gastrointest Endosc 16:11–17, 1969.

17. Rodney WM, Quan MA, Johnson RA, Beaber RJ: Impact of flexible sigmoidoscopy on physician compliance with colorectal cancer screening protocol. J Family Prac 15:885–889, 1982.

18. Salmon R, Branch RA, Collins C, et al.: Clinical evaluation of fibreoptic sigmoidoscopy employing the Olympus CF–SB colonoscope. Gut 12:729–735, 1971.

19. Synder DN, Hester JF, Meigs JW, et al.: Changes in site distribution of colorectal carcinoma in Connecticut, 1940–1973. Am J Dig Dis 22:791–797, 1977.

20. Turell R: Fiber optic coloscope and sigmoidoscope. Am J Surg 105:133–136, 1963.

21. Turell R: Examination, in Turell R (Ed): Diseases of the Colon and Rectum, Vol 1. Philadelphia, WB Saunders, 1969, p 188.

22. Winawer SJ, Leidner SD, Boyle C, Kurtz RC: Comparison of flexible sigmoidoscopy with other diagnostic techniques in the diagnosis of rectocolon neoplasia. Dig Dis Sci 24:277–281, 1979.

23. Winawer SJ, Cummins R, Baldwin MP, Ptak A: A new flexible sigmoidoscope for the generalist. Gastrointest Endosc 28:233–236, 1982.

24. Wolff WI, Shinya H: Colonofiberoscopy. JAMA 217:1509–1512, 1971.

25. Wolff WI, Shinya H: Polypectomy via the fiberoptic colonoscope. Removal of neoplasms beyond reach of the sigmoidoscope. N Engl J Med 288:329–332, 1973.

26. Wolff WI, Shinya H: The impact of colonoscopy on the problem of colorectal cancer. In Ariel IM (Ed): Progress in Clinical Cancer. New York, Grune and Stratton, 1978, pp 51–69.

27. Zucker GM, Madura MJ, Chmiel JS, Olinger EJ: The advantages of the 30-cm flexible sigmoidoscope over the 60-cm flexible sigmoidscope. Gastrointest Endosc 30:59–64, 1984.

2

Fiberscopes: History, Optical and Mechanical
Principles, and Maintenance

The development of fiber optics and the application of this technology to endoscopy has led to major advances in the diagnosis and therapy of diseases in many organ systems. The impact of fiberscopes on the management of diseases of the gastrointestinal tract has been particularly striking. Pathology located in the esophagus, stomach, duodenum, biliary tree, pancreas, and colon can now be accurately identified. Moreover, conditions such as gastrointestinal and colonic polyps, foreign bodies, and common duct stones, to name a few, can now be treated via fiberscopes with significantly less patient morbidity and lower cost.

In this chapter the discovery and historical development of fiber optics will be briefly reviewed, and the optical and general mechanical principles of fiberscopes outlined. Finally, guidelines for the care and maintenance of fiberscopes will be discussed.

HISTORICAL DEVELOPMENT OF FIBEROPTICS

The history of endoscopic visualization of the colon by sigmoidoscopy is reviewed in some detail in Chapter 1. In the first part of this chapter, the historical development of fiber optics and the application of this technology to endoscopy in general and sigmoidoscopy in particular is outlined.

Endoscopic Illumination Prior to Fiberoptics

Prior to the advent of fiberoptic endoscopy, inspection of the upper and lower gastrointestinal tract was limited by inferior optics and rigid instruments (Fig. 2-1A). The first practical endoscopes were straight

Conventional open tube endoscope   Light source

Conventional telescope (Nitze)   Light source
                                     Lens   Air

Rod lens telescope (Hopkins)   Light source
                                     Air   Lens

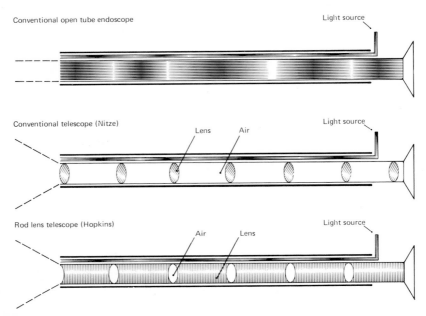

Figure 2-1. Standard methods of endoscopic illumination other than fiber optics. Modified from Gans SL: Principles of optics and illumination. In Gans SL (Ed): Pediatric Endoscopy. New York, Grune & Stratton, 1983, p 3.

metal tubes with various types of primitive light sources, such as reflected candle light.[9] An important development in illumination was the utilization of an electric light source at the proximal and distal end of an open endoscope.[3] A major advance in endoscopic optics occurred when Nitze in 1879 developed a telescope consisting of several small lenses placed at intervals with air spaces in between the lenses (Fig. 2-1B).[3] The system developed by Nitze was first applied to cystoscopy but became the standard optical system for all endoscopy for many years. The final advance in illumination that revolutionized rigid telescopes was the invention by Hopkins of a rod lens optical system for telescopes.[3] In the Hopkins system a series of long glass rods with the ends shaped in the form of a lens are placed in sequence, with small air spaces between the concave ends of adjacent rods (Fig. 2-1C). This system provided an expanded field of view, much improved light transmission, and good optical resolution.

Discovery of Fiberoptics

The modern era of endoscopy dawned in 1954 when Hopkins and Kapany reported in *Nature* the development of a new optical unit they termed a *fiberscope*.[7] Their unit was comprised of a 4-inch bundle of fine glass fibers which would convey optical images along a flexible axis. Prior to their publication, the idea of conveying images along flexible glass fibers had been proposed in 1927 by Baird in a British patent specification[7] and actually accomplished by Lamm in 1930.[10] However, Hopkins and Kapany engineered the first prototype flexible endoscope that could be easily bent without deterioration of the image quality.

Application of Fiberoptics to Gastrointestinal Endoscopy

The transition of fiber optics from theory to practice involved the collaboration of two physicists, Peters and Curtiss, and a gastroenterologist, Hirschowitz, at the University of Michigan.[6] Hirschowitz visited Hopkins and Kapany soon after their description of a fiberscope in 1956 and then began developing a gastroscope. He and his colleagues in physics encountered a number of technical problems, of which the most troublesome was *crosstalk*—the loss of light and image from one fiber to another when fibers are in close contact. However, by December 1956 Curtiss solved the problem of optical insulation of the glass fibers in the bundle by coating each fiber with a thin exterior layer of additional glass of a lower refractive index. This major optical advance led to the production in 6 weeks of the first fiberoptic gastroscope, which was initially swallowed by Hirschowitz himself and then passed into the stomach of the first patient in February 1957. The initial clinical experience with this original fiberoptic gastroscope was published a year later.[5]

Fiberoptic Examination of the Colon

The first attempts at fiberoptic examination of the colon were made with modified gastrocameras and prototype colonoscopes in Japan between 1963–65.[16] The left colon was also visualized with existing fiberoptic gastroscopes.[11] Overholt was the first to study fiberoptic sigmoidoscopy in the United States, with relatively crude original instruments manufactured by several companies, and reported his initial experience between 1968–71.[12–14] He employed several different instruments but reported his largest early experience with the 86-cm Olympus colonofiberscope, short bundle (CF–SB) and 105-cm ACMI instruments that permitted tip deflection in one plane only.[14] Fiberoptic instruments for examination of the entire colon were rapidly made available and the techniques of insertion improved to allow visualization all the way to the cecum.[2] Wolff and Shinya soon reported their extensive experience with the 186-cm colonofiberscope (Olympus CF–LB) for accurate diagnosis of pathology of the entire colon and safe performance of polypectomy by snare cautery.[17–18] Colonoscopy is now an established procedure in standard gastrointestinal practice by specialists, but sigmoidoscopy continues to be performed by generalists with variable instruments, most often the rigid open sigmoidoscope. As discussed elsewhere in this book, 60-cm and 35-cm fiberoptic sigmoidoscopes were developed between 1976–82 and are being increasingly employed by general practitioners in their routine practice, particularly as comparative studies demonstrate their superiority over the rigid instrument.

OPTICAL AND MECHANICAL PRINCIPLES OF FIBERSCOPES

Principles of Fiber Optics

The optical principles that underlie the mechanism of light and image transmission by fiberoptic endoscopes are outlined succinctly in recent endoscopic texts[3,15] and in more detail in several publications.[1,4,7,8] Fiberoptic endoscopes transmit light into the lumen and return images via bundles composed of thousands of fine glass threads 5–25 microns in diameter. Each individual glass fiber in a bundle can transmit light entering at a critical angle of incidence by a process of internal reflection (Fig. 2-2). Loss of light or image transmission is reduced by coating each glass fiber with a thin layer of another type of glass, which has a lower refractive index. These thin glass fibers not only transmit light and images but also are flexible without loss of the angle of incidence of the light ray. The arrangement of thousands of fibers with the above characteristics into a single bundle forms the basic operational feature of a flexible fiberoptic endoscope.

Fiberoptic bundles may be employed for two basic purposes in gastrointestinal endoscopes (1) transmission of light from a proximal light source to illuminate the intestinal lumen; and (2) transport of an image from the lumen back to the proximal portion of endoscope (Fig. 2-3).[15] In the light-transmitting or incoherent bundle, no precise alignment of fibers is necessary and fibers of 25 microns are generally employed. The light that issues from the distal end of the glass fibers is cold, in contrast to the external high-intensity light source which is hot. The fibers in the image-transmitting or coherent bundle must be aligned so that individual fibers bear the same spatial relationship at both ends of

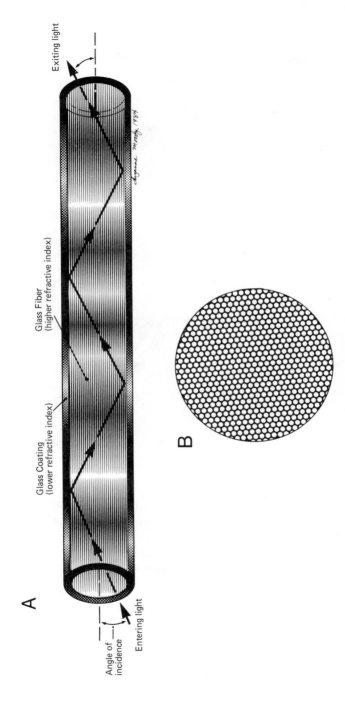

Figure 2-2. Schematic representation of (**A**) transmission of light along individual glass fiber and (**B**) end surface of fiberoptic bundle containing thousands of individual fibers.

13

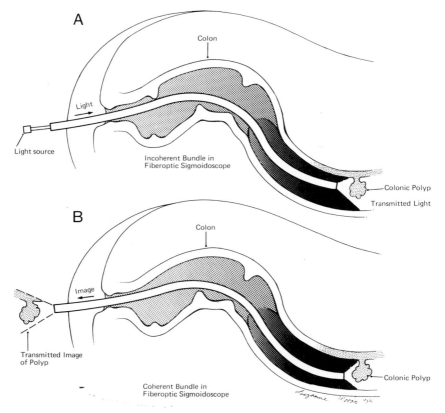

Figure 2-3. Schematic representation of **(A)** light-transmitting or incoherent bundle in a flexible sigmoidoscope and **(B)** image-transmitting or coherent bundle.

the bundle. The coherent bundle consists of 15,000–75,000 nearly identical fibers that are somewhat smaller than in the incoherent bundle. The actual image resolution of individual manufacturer's fiberscopes depends upon several characteristics of the glass fibers such as fiber size (smaller size = better resolution), correctness of their orientation, density, and compactness.

Mechanics of Endoscopes

The construction of modern endoscopes is very complex. Only the mechanical features common to all endoscopes will be presented in very general and schematic terms. Details regarding the specifications

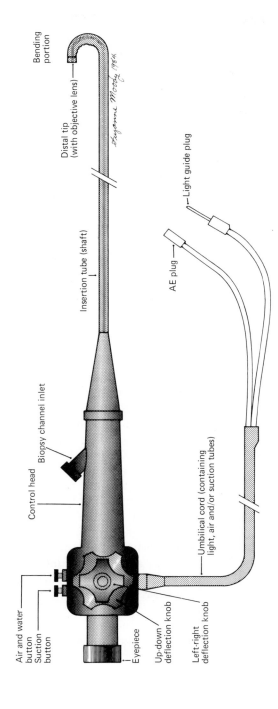

Air and water
button
Suction
button

Eyepiece

Up-down
deflection knob

Left-right
deflection knob

Control head

Biopsy channel inlet

Umbilical cord (containing
light, air and/or suction tubes)

Insertion tube (shaft)

Distal tip
(with objective lens)

Bending
portion

AE plug

Light guide plug

Figure 2-4. Nomenclature of standard fiberoptic sigmoidoscope.

15

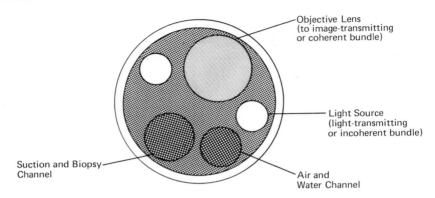

Figure 2-5. Fiberoptic tip details of a standard instrument (American ACMI).

of flexible sigmoidoscopes currently produced by five manufacturers are reviewed in Chapter 5.

The typical fiberoptic sigmoidoscope with the nomenclature of its functional parts is shown in Figure 2-4. The basic instrument consists of a control head, a flexible insertion tube (shaft), and a maneuverable tip. The control head is attached to a connecting (umbilical) cord containing tubes that transmit light, air, and/or suction from external sources. Hidden within the insertion tube of the endoscope are the most important functional elements—the fiberoptic bundles. Each end of the fiberoptic bundles is polished, and the coherent bundle is fitted with a series of lenses.[15] A distal or objective lens is needed to focus the image of the object to be viewed on the plane of the distal bundle. This image is inverted and transmitted to the proximal end of the bundle, where it is restored to normal orientation, magnified and focused by a proximal lens or eyepiece.

In addition to fiber bundles for light and image transmission, the standard fiberscope has proximal control knobs and wires along its length to permit deflection of the distal bending portion and tip in both the up–down and left–right directions. An open channel is built into the instrument to allow suction, an important function of flexible sigmoidoscopes, and passage of biopsy and other diagnostic and therapeutic instruments. Another smaller channel allows insufflation of air, to distend the lumen, and water to wash the distal tip (Fig. 2-5). The suction and air/water buttons are located on top of the control head at a proximal site, and the biopsy channel inlet is usually placed slightly more distal on the control head. The exterior of the fiberscope is usually encased by circumferential metal braids and covered with a durable plastic sheath.

CARE AND MAINTENANCE OF FIBERSCOPES

Proper care and maintenance of fiberscopes is an essential owner-ship component of these relatively expensive instruments. A fiberoptic endoscope is a delicate optical instrument, and its useful life may be shortened by improper care and handling. Each instrument has its own operating and maintenance manual that should be read and studied thoroughly. Careful review of the manual is also a good investment, since manufacturers estimate that more than 50% of repairs are neces-sitated by improper care or maintenance.

Protocols for general care, cleaning, disinfection, and storage should be established in the office or hospital where the instrument is used. In larger endoscopic units, gastrointestinal assistants and nurses are trained in proper cleaning and maintenance of fiberoptic endoscopes; however, physicians and other endoscopists must be familiar with proper usage to maintain fiberscope durability. In smaller units or offices, cleaning and maintenance is best standardized by training and assigning respon-sibility to a single individual.

General Precautions

The following general precautions apply to the use to of fiberscopes:

1. Endoscopy should be performed only by persons with ade-quate training and after review of appropriate medical litera-ture.
2. The instruction manual accompanying the fiberscope should be studied in detail.
3. Verify that the instrument functions properly (e.g., light, air, water, control knobs) before each use. Do not use if fiberscope is malfunctioning or the covering of the shaft is broken.
4. Do not deflect the distal shaft sharply by hand.
5. Do not bend the insertion tube or light guide sharply.
6. Do not allow the distal tip to come in sharp contact with any hard object.
7. Avoid forceful and rapid manipulation of the tip deflection control knobs.
8. Do not immerse or splash fluid on the control head, which is generally not water-tight.
9. Do not steam autoclave the fiberscopes.
10. Avoid unnecessary exposure of the fiberscope to x-rays.
11. Be familiar with biopsy and polypectomy instruments before use.

12. Do not force any accessory instrument through the biopsy channel.
13. Clean immediately after use (see below).

Cleaning and Disinfection

Cleaning is important to prevent damage to the instrument channels—and other parts of the fiberscope—from dried materials, and disinfection is necessary to destroy potential infective organisms. Cleaning and disinfection are best combined into one procedure after each use of the instrument.

The term disinfection and sterilization are often confused and used interchangeably. Disinfection is the destruction of all infective organisms except spores and is achieved by a number of commercially available chemical solutions. Sterilization is the ultimate form of disinfection and is defined by the destruction of all types of infective agents, including bacteria, fungi, viruses, and spores. Many of the commercial disinfecting solutions will destroy spores and thus sterilize the instrument, but the prolonged contact time required (3–24 hours) makes sterilization not practical on a routine basis. Most flexible sigmoidoscopes can be disinfected with 10–30 minutes exposure to several preparations, such as 70% alcohol (disinfectant ethanol), povidone–iodine (Betadine), iodophor (e.g., Wescodyne) or glutaraldehyde (e.g., Sporicidin, Cidex). The manufacturer's instruction manuals should be consulted to confirm the compatibility of these chemical solutions with the instrument materials. In routine practice, one of the various glutaraldehyde preparations are usually employed for disinfection. Most instruments have also been designed to be sterilized by ethylene oxide gas as an alternative to chemical disinfection. Gas sterilization is too expensive and takes too long (24 hours) to be practical for routine use. It is usually employed in special situations when absolute sterility is desired, e.g., before endoscopy in immunosuppressed or severely neutropenic patients and after endoscopy in patients with hepatitis B or acquired immune deficiency syndrome (AIDS).

The manual washing and disinfection procedure for each instrument is clearly outlined in the manufacturer's instruction manual accompanying the flexible sigmoidoscope. Mechanical cleaning with soap and water is a critically important first step that permits chemical disinfection to be effective. The general approach to cleaning and disinfection of flexible sigmoidoscopes is as follows:

1. The exterior of the endoscope is washed with warm detergent and gauze pads, taking care to keep the control head dry.

2. A cleaning brush is then run through the biopsy channel, and detergent aspirated through the suction channel.
3. The biopsy channel inlet on the control head is removed, cleaned, and reassembled.
4. The insertion tube is then placed in disinfectant, which is also aspirated into the suction channel and left in place for 2–20 minutes.
5. Disinfectant is also flushed through the air/water channels.
6. The instrument is then removed from disinfectant, and the insertion tube and all channels are rinsed with water.
7. The instrument is then air dried by wiping the shaft, injection of air by syringe through the biopsy channel, and operation of the air button.

Most endoscopic units clean and disinfect their instruments manually, but automated cleaning units (e.g., System 83 by Custom Ultrasonic, Automatic Endoscope Cleaner Model 187 by American Endoscopy Inc.) are available. In the automated system, the endoscope shaft is placed in position with the control head secured outside the interior wash chamber. A pulsating pump is attached to the endoscope channels, which are cleaned by a series of washes. The channels are first flushed with water at 105°F, washed with a detergent, rinsed again with hot water, disinfected with a cold sterilizing solution, and then rinsed with water a final time before dried with air. The advantage of the automated unit is that it frees the gastrointestinal assistant to spend more time with patients or at other duties. The major disadvantage of these automatic endoscope washers is their cost, which averages $8,000–12,000.

Cleaning and disinfection is modified in a few special situations. Patients who are severely neutropenic or immunocompromised should ideally undergo sigmoidoscopy with instruments and acessories that have been previously sterilized. The risk of hepatitis B transmission by flexible sigmoidoscopy is very remote, and meticulous attention to mechancial washing and disinfection is probably all that is required following procedures on these patients. Flexible sigmoidoscopes and accessories used to examine patients with AIDS should be mechanically washed with copious amounts of detergent and ideally be gas sterilized or at least undergo prolonged chemical disinfection. Personnel involved in sigmoidoscopy of these patients should wear gloves and gowns during the procedure and instrument clean-up.

Storage

Most instrument manuals recommend vertical storage on a hanger or wall rack to promote drainage. Wall racks should be engineered such that the fiberscope is securely mounted to prevent an inadvertent fall when a nearby fiberscope is removed. The sigmoidoscope carrying case should only be employed for long-term storage or transportation from one place to another.

REFERENCES

 1. Bird EW: Fibre optics. A current appraisal. Med Biol Ill 12:167–173, 1962.
 2. Dean ACB, Shearman DJC: Clinical evaluation of a new fibreoptic colonoscope. Lancet 1:550–552, 1970.
 3. Gans SL: Principle of optics and illumination, in Gans SL (Ed): Pediatric Endoscopy. New York, Grune & Stratton, 1983, pp 1–8.
 4. Hirschowitz BI: Fibre optics in modern medicine. Med Biol Ill 15:224–229, 1965.
 5. Hirschowitz BI, Curtiss LE, Peters CW, Pollard HM: Demonstration of a new gastroscope, the "fiberscope." Gastroenterology 35:50–53, 1958.
 6. Hirschowitz BI: A personal history of the fiberscope. Gastroenterology 76:864–869, 1979.
 7. Hopkins HH, Kapany NS: A flexible fibrescope, using static scanning. Nature 173:39–41, 1954.
 8. Kapany N: Fibre optics. Scientific American 203:72–81, 1960.
 9. Kelly HDB: Origins of oesophagology. Proc Roy Soc Med 62:781–786, 1969.
10. Lamm H: Biegsame optishe gerate. Z Instrumentenkunde 50:579, 1930.
11. Lemire S, Cocco AE: Visualization of the left colon with the fiber optic gastroduodenoscope. Gastrointest Endosc 13:29–30, 1966.
12. Overholt BF: Clinical experience with the fibersigmoidoscope. Gastrointest Endosc 15:27, 1968.
13. Overholt BF: Flexible fiberoptic sigmoidoscopes. CA 19:81–84, 1969.
14. Overholt BF: Flexible fiberoptic sigmoidoscopy. Technique and preliminary results. Cancer 28:123–126, 1971.
15. Patil VU, Stehling LC, Zauder HL: Fiberoptic Endoscopy in Anesthesia. Chicago: Year Book Medical Publishers, pp 1–7.
16. Sivak MV, Sullivan BH Jr, Rankin GB: Colonoscopy. A report of 644 cases and review of the literature. Am J Surg 128:351–357, 1974.
17. Wolff WI, Shinya H: Colonofiberoscopy. JAMA 217:1509–1512, 1971.
18. Wolff WI, Shinya H: Polypectomy via the fiberoptic colonoscope. Removal of neoplasms beyond reach of the sigmoidoscope. N Engl J Med 288:329–332, 1973.

3
Technique of Flexible Sigmoidoscopy

INSTRUMENT CONTROLS AND THEIR OPERATION

The operator should become thoroughly familiar with all instrument functions before employing the flexible sigmoidoscope in practice. Manufacturer's instruments vary not only in length but also in design and operation of controls for air, water, and suction (see Chapter 5). Instrument control heads are generally arranged in one of two formats (Figs. 3-1 and 3-2). Most models are engineered with four-way tip deflection, but one has only two-way deflection. Proper connection of the instrument to the light source and suction apparatus should be learned, and each function should be routinely checked prior to beginning a procedure. Biopsy, photographic equipment, polypectomy snares, and electrocoagulation apparatus should be in working order and readily accessible.

A period of training with an experienced endoscopist is highly desirable before beginning flexible sigmoidoscopy. Ideally at least 10, and preferably 20 examinations should be performed with a preceptor before beginning independent examinations. Some experience with a colon model and videotapes may also be helpful. The new operator should fully understand the indications, technique, contraindications, and complications of flexible sigmoidoscopy. A review of the photographs illustrating various colonic disorders in Chapter 11 and in published colonoscopy textbooks will improve the accurate visual diagnosis of colonic mucosal abnormalities and pathological lesions.

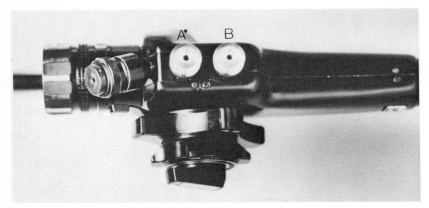

Figure 3-1. Control head. Proximal valve **(A)** produces suction when depressed. Distal valve **(B)** controls air insufflation by touch and water jet when depressed.

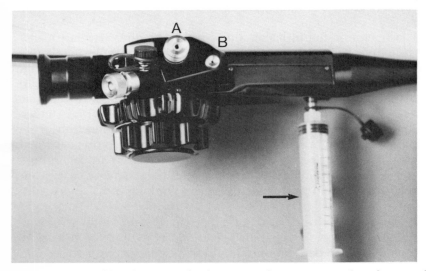

Figure 3-2. Control head. Proximal valve **(A)** produces suction when depressed. Distal valve **(B)** controls air insufflation only. Syringe attached to side port *(arrow)* allows injection of forceful water jet to clear lens of debris.

PATIENT PREPARATION

Psychological Preparation

Good rapport with the patient who is about to undergo flexible sigmoidoscopy is essential and is enhanced by careful explanation of the reasons for the procedure. It may be helpful to show the patient the flexible instrument and demonstrate its maneuverability. The patient should be warned that there may be some discomfort due to air insufflation and bowel stretching and that he or she should alert you if the pain becomes severe, in which case you may discontinue instrument advancement or suction out some of the insufflated air.

Bowel Preparation

An effective bowel preparation must be achieved for optimal visualization at sigmoidoscopy (endoscopic street cleaners and windshield washers are just not adequate in foul colonic conditions!). Most endoscopists employ one or two 4-ounce phosphate enemas (Fleets or Phospho–Soda) prior to the examination, which yields adequate preparation in 80–90% of cases. Some feel that two enemas produce more rectosigmoid effluent from proximal areas and that one enema is preferable. Enemas are usually given 10–20 minutes before the examination is performed, although they may be taken at home 1–2 hours before the procedure. Occasionally, in severely constipated patients, who are often elderly, a full bowel preparation such as those used for barium enema or colonoscopy may be required.

Patients with severe active inflammatory bowel disease should not in general undergo colon preparation since colonic contents are already liquid. In addition, enemas and/or laxatives may increase friability and alter assessment of the disease activity or may actually be harmful and result in increased bleeding, distention, or perforation. If the activity of the colitis is only mild to moderate, a single gentle tap water enema may be used.

SEDATION

Sedation for flexible sigmoidoscopy, as with rigid sigmoidoscopy, is rarely necessary. Apprehensive patients can usually be reassured that the procedure will not produce severe pain and will only last a few minutes. During the procedure, verbal tranquilization should be provided by reassuring the patient and keeping him or her appraised of the progress of the examination. Small amounts of intravenous diazepam may be required for patients with extreme apprehension, severe perianal disease or painful hemorrhoids, and also for children.

POSITIONING OF PATIENT (LEFT LATERAL VERSUS INVERTED)

The ideal patient position for flexible sigmoidoscopy is a matter of examiner preference. Studies in the literature are divided between use of the inverted (Fig. 3-3) or left lateral (Sims) positions (Fig. 3-4). Patient tolerance is probably similar with either position. The inverted position on a standard sigmoidoscopic tilt table is favored by some because (1) this position is more familiar to the new operator who previously performed rigid sigmoidoscopy in this position; (2) the examination of the perianal region and anal canal is easier; and (3) the table can be tilted down easily should the patient have a vasovagal episode. The sigmoidoscopic table need not be tipped down more than 15–20°. The extreme head down position ("jackknife") used for rigid sigmoidoscopy is not necessary for flexible sigmoidoscopy.

Many physicians practicing in offices and small clinics do not own or have easy access to an expensive sigmoidoscopic tilt table. Purchase of such a table is not necessary for adequate performance of flexible sigmoidoscopy. In fact, many experienced endoscopists favor the left

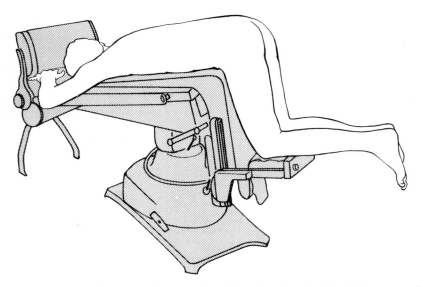

Figure 3-3. Inverted position. Patient should be tipped only 15°–20° downward on the tilt table.

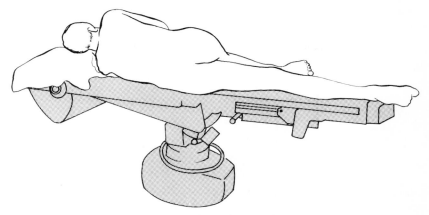

Figure 3-4. Left lateral (Sims) position.

lateral (Sims) position because (1) this position is routinely used for colonoscopy, and the examiner is more familiar with sigmoid colon landmarks and insertion maneuvers in this position; (2) certain patients with limited mobility (e.g., pregnancy, ascites, severe arthritis, fracture, marked weakness, and debility) are more comfortable in this position; and (3) the lateral position is convenient for bedside examination of hospitalized patients.

PERIANAL INSPECTION

A thorough inspection of the perianal area should be accomplished before actual sigmoidoscopy. The examiner should routinely look for evidence of hemorrhoids (i.e., size, ulceration, thrombosis), fissures and fistulae (location, drainage), rectal prolapse, and specific pathologic processes such as chancres, condylomata, herpetic vesicles, etc.

ANOSCOPY

Examination of the anal canal (Fig. 3-5) should be a routine part of every sigmoidoscopic examination. Patients with symptoms localized to the anus (i.e., pain, burning, itching) should undergo anoscopy before sigmoidoscopy. This examination can be performed with a standard metal anoscope. However, this separate procedure is not routinely necessary, since most anal pathology can be well seen with the flexible sigmoidoscope by insufflation of air in the anal canal during careful,

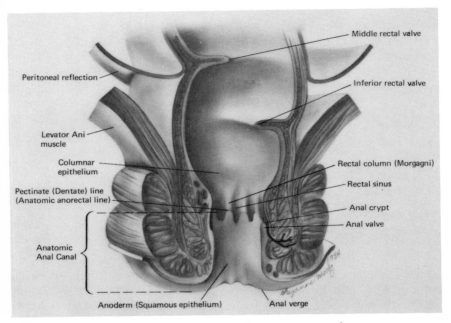

Figure 3-5. Sagittal section of lower rectum and anus.

slow withdrawal. Routine search for internal hemorrhoids, anal fissures, cryptitis, and anal cancer should be performed. Inexperienced examiners often neglect the anal canal during flexible sigmoidoscopy by removing the instrument too rapidly from the distal rectum rather than slowly removing the sigmoidoscope and carefully inspecting the anal canal.

INSERTION OF THE FLEXIBLE SIGMOIDOSCOPE

Rectal examination with a well-lubricated gloved finger should always be performed prior to insertion of the sigmoidoscope. The purpose of this maneuver is to (1) relax the rectal sphincter and prelubricate the anal canal; (2) detect pathology in the anal canal, rectum, and prostate; (3) detect gross or occult blood, pus, or mucus; and (4) confirm that the rectum has been adequately cleared of feces.

The distal 10–15 cm of the sigmoidoscope should be lubricated with a suitable jelly. Lubricants containing local anesthetics can be employed when active anal disease is present. One should take care not to lubricate the sigmoidoscope tip, since lubricants will cloud the lens and obscure vision.

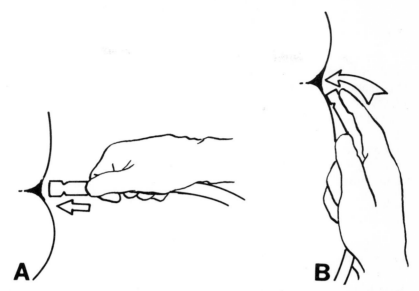

Figure 3-6. Insertion technique: **(A)** Incorrect; 180° direct insertion. **(B)** Correct; 90° *wedged* insertion.

Since the tip of the instrument is blunt, a straight 180° end-on insertion should not be attempted (Fig. 3-6A). This approach may result in discomfort, increase patient anxiety, and even cause an anal abrasion or tear. Proper insertion consists of placing the forefinger parallel on the surface of the instrument and entering the anus from a 90° right-angle approach (Fig. 3-6B). The patient can be instructed to bear down during insertion to help relax the anal sphincter. An alternative inser-tion technique is to substitute the sigmoidoscope tip for the examining finger during withdrawal from digital examination.

CONTROL OF INSERTION TUBE AND TIP DEFLECTION

Once the tip of the flexible sigmoidoscope is inserted into the rectum, the operator can choose a one-person or two-person technique to control advancement of the insertion tube or shaft.

One-Person versus Two-Person Technique

One-person technique   The instrument head is supported by the left hand, which is cupped with the thumb around the base to control the deflection knobs while the fingers are free to work the valves on top of the instrument (Fig. 3-7). The insertion (pushing) can be accomplished with the examiner's free right hand (Fig. 3-8).

Two-person technique   The instrument is held in the cupped left hand with the fingers free to control the valves for air, water, and suction. This leaves the right hand free to control the tip deflection knobs (Fig. 3-9). With this technique, an assistant must be available to hold the shaft of the instrument and gently advance as directed by the endoscopist. It is very helpful if the assistant views the colon via a teaching attachment during advancement (Fig. 3-10). This two-person technique utilizing a teaching attachment is useful to teach new examiners anatomic landmarks, insertion technique, and interpretative skills.

Tip Deflection

An instrument with 4-way tip deflection capability is preferable for easy advancement of the sigmoidoscope through the colon. The degree of up–down and left–right tip deflection of the different models of sigmoidoscopes is variable (see Chapter 5). Downward rotation of the large control knob directs the tip downward 170–180°, while upward rotation deflects the instrument tip upwards to the same degree. Downward rotation of the small control knob moves the tip to the right 140°–180° and upward rotation causes leftward tip deflection to a similar degree (Fig. 3-11).

Several points should be kept in mind when operating the control knobs to achieve successful and safe tip deflection. The control knobs should be turned slowly. Rapid tip deflection causes undue patient discomfort and stresses the instrument cables, which can lead to damage and expensive repair bills. The least degree of flexion necessary to visualize the lumen should be used. Instrument advancement is more difficult when the tip is sharply angled. A tight angle may in effect become a leading edge, resulting in little force actually reaching the instrument tip. In general, both up-down and left-right control knobs should not be used at the same time. Finally, after tip deflection has located the lumen, the instrument should be advanced a short way and then the tip returned to a neutral position.

AIR INSUFFLATION

The least amount of air insufflation required to maintain an open lumen is most desirable in performing flexible sigmoidoscopy. Excessive air insufflation causes spasm, colonic distention, and patient discomfort. In addition, overenthusiastic use of air may create a large

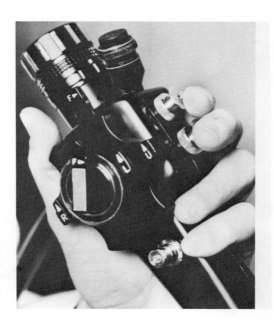

Figure 3-7. One-person technique. Examiner controls valves with index and third finger of left hand, while thumb works the directional control dial.

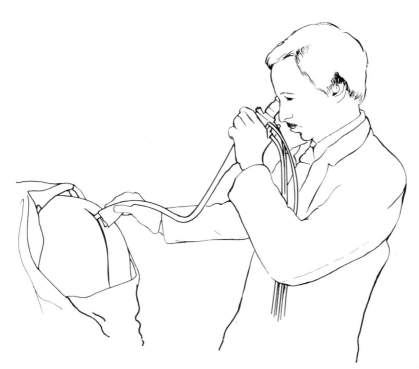

Figure 3-8. One-person technique. Examiner's free right hand controls insertion tube by pushing and torque.

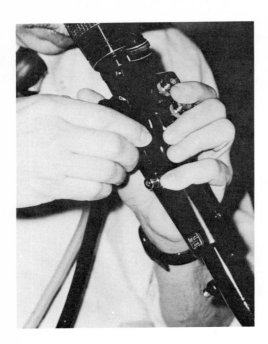

Figure 3-9. Two-person technique. Examiner's right hand works the directional control dials, while left hand operates valves for suction, air, and water.

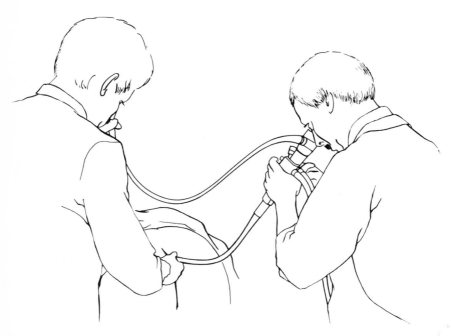

Figure 3-10. Two-person technique. Primary examiner has both hands on the control head and a second examiner advances and torques insertion tube, while viewing through *lecturescope*.

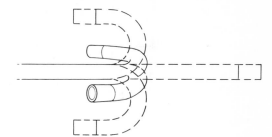

Figure 3-11. 4-way directional tip control.

sigmoid loop, increase the acuteness of the sigmoid-descending colon junction, and make instrument insertion more difficult. The colon is elastic, and thus it may become elongated and tortuous when inflated. When it is deflated, the colon becomes shorter and often more receptive to passage of the sigmoidoscope. Overinsufflation can also cause perforation of a diverticulum, serosal lacerations, or pneumatic perforation of the cecum (see Chapter 9).

ANORECTAL VISUALIZATION

Anal Canal

Tip deflection cannot be accomplished in the anal canal due to external pressure of the anal sphincter muscle. When the rectum is entered, a slight "give" will be felt. The anal canal is best visualized during withdrawal of the instrument.

Rectum

After passing through the anal canal, the first view may be a red-out or a blurred view of liquid contents. A red-out indicates that the lens is against the mucosa and the instrument needs to be pulled back slightly. Gentle air insufflation and suction of liquid contents should make the rectum clearly visible. Use suction in short bursts. Suction of long duration will be ineffective since it will "suck up" mucosa. It may also create erythematous, circular marks (*artifacts*), which may be mistaken for small polyps. Do not attempt suction of solid or semi-solid stool, since it will be ineffective and result in clogging the suction channel. Temporary clogging of the lens by mucus or stool can often be handled by simply passing the biopsy forceps down the open channel. If the preparation is very poor, discontinue the procedure and give the patient another cleansing enema or repeat the procedure on another day.

The normal mucosa with a glistening salmon-pink surface and branching vascular pattern should be visible (see Chapter 11, Fig. 11-1). Any lesions observed during advancement of the endoscope should be noted, although a more detailed visualization is usually accomplished on withdrawal. The shaft should, in general, only be advanced when the colonic lumen is identified. Usually the lumen is easily followed in the distended rectum. The three valves of Houston, which are prominent haustral folds, will be clearly seen (Fig. 3–12). Occasionally, inadvertent retroflexion may occur, and the shaft can be visualized in the distal rectum and anus (See Chapter 11, Figure 11-2). A clue that retroflexion is occurring is increased patient discomfort associated with poor instrument advancement. Retroflexion can be corrected by straightening the tip, pulling the scope back slightly, and locating the lumen again before advancing. Some examiners advocate the retroflexion maneuver as an integral part of the examination to better visualize the distal rectum.

SIGMOID AND DESCENDING COLON VISUALIZATION

Upon entering the sigmoid colon, the haustral pattern becomes more evident, the lumen narrows, and several sharp angulations must be negotiated. It is in the sigmoid colon that the examiner earns his or her "stripes."

Luminal Visualization

A direct luminal or *tunnel view* may be obvious in certain areas of the sigmoid colon, but it is most common in the descending colon (Fig. 3-13). If the lumen cannot be identified, it is preferable not to proceed blindly. It is better to pull the tip back a few centimeters and look for one of several clues.[2,3,6] The mucosa near the lumen will be darker, since it is further away from the endoscope tip illumination (Fig. 3-14). The lumen will be around a sharp bend if an arc of mucosa is seen against a shadowed background (Fig. 3-15). It may be helpful to use both gentle torque of the shaft along with minimal tip deflection to negotiate such

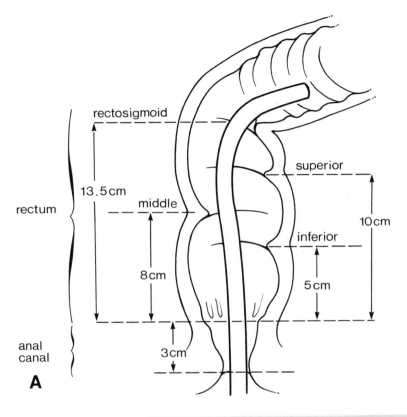

rectosigmoid

13.5 cm

rectum

middle

superior

10 cm

inferior

8 cm

5 cm

anal
canal

3 cm

A

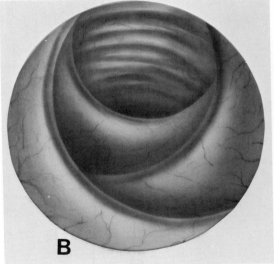

B

Figure 3-12. The rectum: **(A)** Sagittal section of rectum showing inferior, middle, and superior valves of Houston and rectosigmoid angle. **(B)** Foreshortened luminal view showing sharp-edged valves of Houston and a normal mucosal vascular pattern.

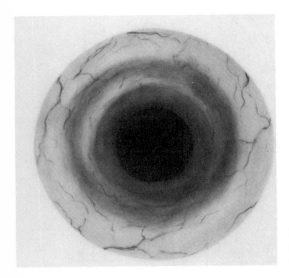

Figure 3-13. Direct luminal ("tunnel") view often seen in descending colon.

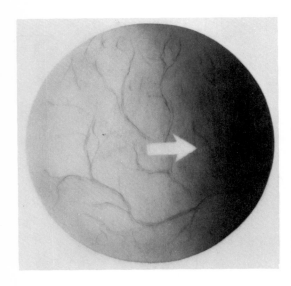

Figure 3-14. The luminal side is further from the light and is therfore darker (*arrow*).

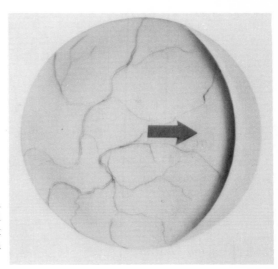

Figure 3-15. An arc of mucosa adjacent to a thin, shadowed background. Lumen lies just beneath arc of mucosa at an acute angle *(arrow)*.

a sharp turn. When the colon is deflated or in spasm, the lumen will be at the center of convergence of the folds (Fig. 3-16). Gentle air insufflation may allow better luminal visualization. For severe spasm, 0.5–1 mg of glucagon given intravenously may be helpful. Look for the concave arcs of the haustral folds. Following their path usually will lead to the

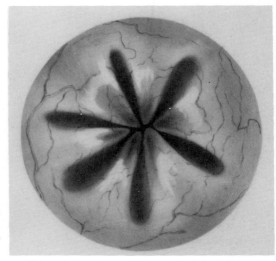

Figure 3-16. Colonic spasm has caused mucosa to pucker. The luman lies in the center of converging folds.

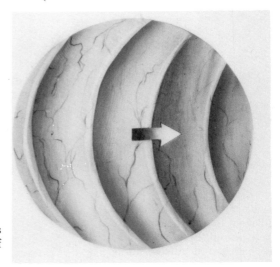

Figure 3-17. The lumen is towards the concave arcs of the haustral folds *(arrow)*.

lumen (Fig. 3-17). When multiple diverticula are present, a large diverticulum may be mistaken for the *lumen*. Careful observation can usually ascertain the actual lumen by noting the presence of haustral folds in normal colon and absence of same in a diverticulum (Fig. 3-18), or the passage of luminal contents.

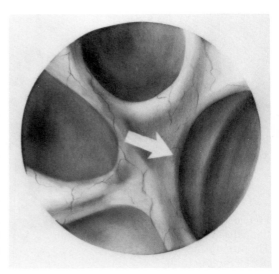

Figure 3-18. Multiple diverticular orifices. Note true lumen with its haustral folds *(arrow)*.

Special Maneuvers for Advancement

The following description of special maneuvers is a synthesis of several reports[2,3,6] as well as our own experience over the last 8 years. Advancement simply by pushing the shaft of the sigmoidoscope is often quite effective, particularly in the rectum and distal sigmoid colon. Simple pushing may not result in advancement of the tip, however, once the redundant middle and proximal sigmoid is reached. Unlike the rectum and descending colon, which are fixed in their position, the sigmoid is mobile on its mesentery. Thus a large sigmoid loop may be formed by upward stretching of the sigmoid colon when the instrument tip is deflected sharply at the sigmoid-descending colon junction but does not advance with further insertion of the instrument shaft. This pattern is called the N-loop (Fig. 3-19) and is a common cause of abdominal distention and pain. The examiner often becomes frustrated because the tip refuses to budge despite good luminal visualization. Early colonscopists found, to their amazement and chagrin, that they could insert

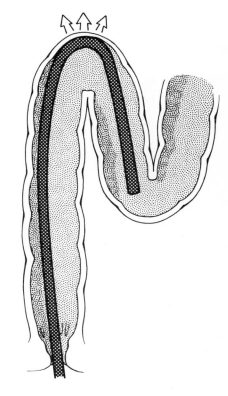

Figure 3-19. The N-loop. This is caused by the upward bowing of the mobile sigmoid colon by the sigmoidoscope. There is now a hairpin sigmoid-descending colon angle, and most of the advancing force is diverted to the deflecting section (arrows) rather than to the tip of the sigmoidoscope.

much of the colonoscope shaft into a patient, only to discover at fluoroscopy that the entire shaft was still in the sigmoid colon. When
advancement of the tip is unsuccessful by simple pushing, a number of
useful techniques can be employed.

Intubation by elongation   At times gentle steady pushing will allow
tip advancement, particularly if the deflected tip angle is somewhat
opened (Fig. 3-20). When further pushing produces blanching of the
mucosa, termed a *white-out,* the instrument should be pulled back a
few centimeters.

Shaft torque   The shaft of the flexible sigmoidoscope is extremely
responsive to external torque by simply rotating the control head of the
instrument or by rotating the shaft itself, near its entrance into the anal

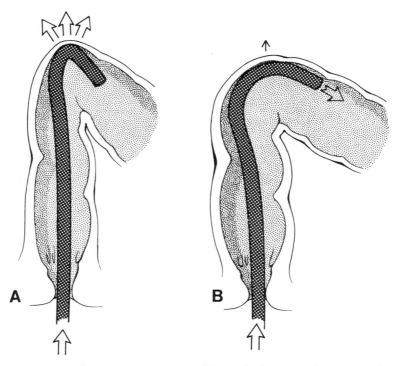

Figure 3-20. Intubation by elongation. **(A)** Marked tip angulation into the sigmoid colon results in the deflecting section becoming the leading edge *(arrows).*
(B) Flattening the deflecting angle allows most of the force to be transmitted to
tip *(large arrows).*

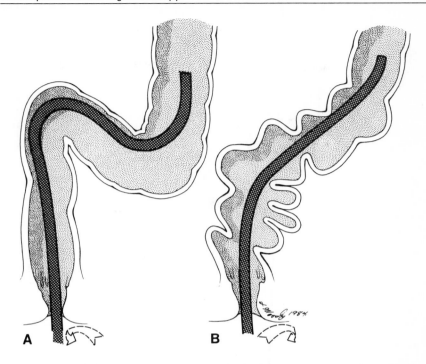

Figure 3-21. Shaft torque. **(A)** Counterclockwise torque (*curved arrow*) has resulted in a markedly curved and stretched sigmoid. The sigmoidoscope is bowed and little force can be directed to the tip. **(B)** Clockwise torque (*curved arrow*) causes the sigmoidoscope to straighten and the sigmoid colon to be *pleated*, allowing tip advancement. For best effect, this maneuver is performed simultaneously with pull-back maneuver (see Figure 3-22).

canal. Counterclockwise torque (Fig. 3-21A) tends to put a bend in the sigmoidoscope and elongate the colon, and should generally be avoided. Gentle clockwise torque of the instrument shaft is an important maneuver for two reasons. First, it is frequently more effective to find and enter a sharply angulated lumen by torquing the gently deflected tip toward the lumen rather than searching and sharply angulating the tip into the lumen. Secondly, when the lumen is well visualized, but tip advancement is not occurring, clockwise torque will usually straighten a curved sigmoidoscope and pleat or *accordionize* the sigmoid onto the sigmoidoscope (Fig. 3-21B). This maneuver is usually more effective when performed as part of the pull-back maneuver (Fig. 3-22).

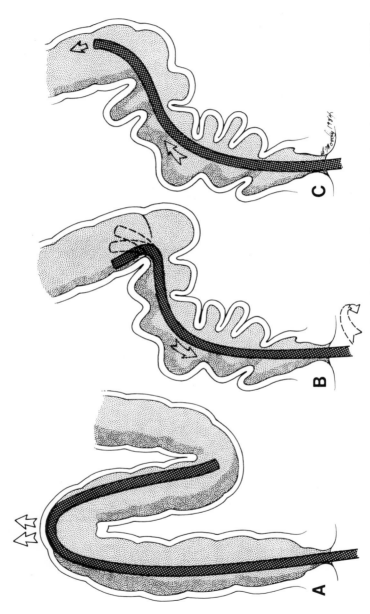

Figure 3-22. Pull-back maneuver. **(A)** An *N-loop* has formed resulting in poor tip advancement. **(B)** The sigmoidoscope tip hooks a haustral fold and the examiner gently pulls the shaft backwards several centimeters (*arrow*). Clockwise torque may also be employed during the pull-back maneuver (*curved, dashed arrow*). **(C)** The sigmoid is *pleated* and the sigmoidoscope tip can now be easily advanced into the descending colon (*arrows*).

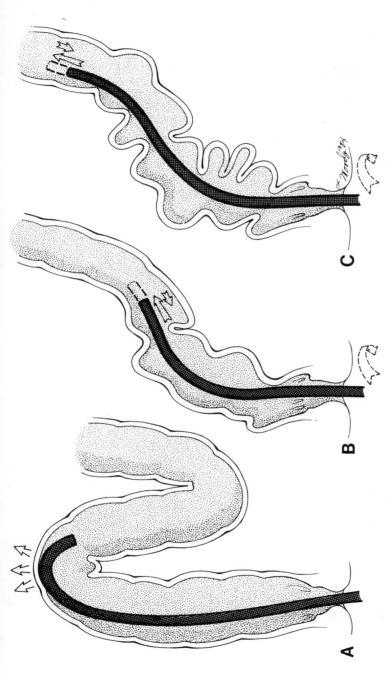

Figure 3-23. Dithering (to-and-fro maneuver). **(A)** Sigmoid loop has developed resulting in force being applied to bending section only (arrows). **(B)** Rapid gentle to-and-fro oscillation (parallel arrows) begins to pleat sigmoid. Counterclockwise torque may also be applied (curved, dashed arrow). **(C)** Continued to-and-fro oscillation (parallel arrows) has resulted in marked pleating and shortening of the sigmoid colon, allowing force to be directed to tip of sigmoidoscope which now enters the descending colon.

Pull-back maneuver   The sigmoidoscope tip can be hooked around a haustral fold and held in that position while the instrument is gently withdrawn several centimeters. This maneuver usually shortens and accordionizes the sigmoid colon on the sigmoidoscope shaft while also eliminating instrument loops. The instrument can then usually be advanced quite easily. This maneuver can be accompanied by clockwise torque (Figure 3-22). It may need to be employed more than once during the procedure.

Dithering   This maneuver involves gentle repetitive 2–3 cm to-and-fro movements of the shaft. Forward motion is rapid, while the withdrawing motion is slower. This technique minimizes the frictional resistance between the colon and the sigmoidoscope and also accordionizes the sigmoid colon onto the sigmoidoscope shaft. It can be employed alone or in combination with clockwise torque (Fig. 3-23).

Slide-by maneuver   In general a luminal view is preferred when advancing the instrument, but occasionally this is not possible. It may be necessary to advance the instrument while the mucosa is seen to freely move *(slide-by)* and the instrument tip clearly advances. After advancing several centimeters, the lumen should be searched for by operation of the tip deflection knobs. Extreme caution should be taken during the slide-by technique, particularly in patients with known diverticular disease, obstructing lesions, and adhesions from previous pelvic surgery.

Other techniques that may be combined with the above maneuvers to reduce sharp sigmoid colon angulation at the sigmoid-descending colon junction include frequent deflation of air to shorten the colon and firm manual pressure over the anterior abdominal wall in the left lower quadrant to reduce the size of instrument loops. If resistence is encountered before full insertion and the above maneuvers fail, attempts at further insertion should be abandoned. Not all patients can undergo safe flexible sigmoidoscopy to full insertion of the instrument. The examiner should be particularly cautious in patients with pelvic adhesions from previous surgery or diverticular disease. The sigmoidoscopist must always weigh the clinical indication for the procedure against the risks of a complication.

WITHDRAWAL OF THE FLEXIBLE SIGMOIDOSCOPE

The best luminal views are obtained on withdrawal of the flexible sigmoidoscope. Withdrawal should be accomplished slowly and carefully, using both tip deflection and torque to visualize in a circumferential fashion as much of the colon as possible. This part of the examination is nearly painless and is well tolerated. Lesions should be carefully studied and their location noted. The location of lesions by notation of the number of centimeters of the instrument inserted is most reliable during withdrawal, after sigmoid loops formed during insertion have been reduced. The mucosal characteristics and location of lesions should be noted at the time of the examination and a complete record dictated or written on a standard procedure form (see Chapter 4).

ENDOSCOPIC BIOPSY

Biopsy forceps that allow for pinch biopsies of mucosa or mass lesions are available and should be regularly employed (Fig. 3-24). The technique for mucosal biopsy is straightforward. The closed forceps are passed slowly and gently down the biopsy channel until they are seen emerging from the tip of the instrument. The assistant is then asked to "open" the biopsy cup. Under direct vision, the forceps are advanced gently but firmly into the tissue that is to be biopsied. The assistant is then instructed to *close* the biopsy cup, and the operator pulls the biopsy cup away from the tissue. If done properly, the tissue will pucker slightly before the cup is pulled away from the tissue. The sample is then put on a grid mesh to aid proper histological orientation and carefully placed in formalin. Multiple biopsies from the same area or lesion are placed in the same container. Biopsies from different areas should be placed in separate containers and each labeled according to the type of lesion

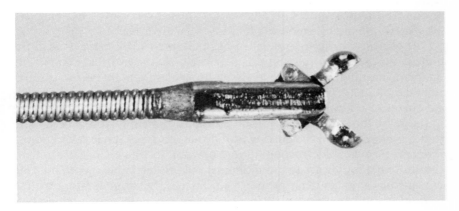

Figure 3-24. Endoscopic biopsy forceps.

and location, e.g., ulcer on base of rectal valve at 8 cm, or ulcerated mass at 28 cm.

The technique of endoscopic pinch biopsy is extremely safe, but certain precautions need to be taken. Biopsy should always be obtained under direct vision. The biopsy forceps should not be pushed forcibly into tissue, particularly inflamed mucosa. If a severe coagulopathy exists, a biopsy may not be safe. Finally, the forceps should always be passed gently through the instrument channel to avoid damage to the forceps or the sigmoidoscope channel.

ENDOSCOPIC POLYPECTOMY

In general polypectomy is performed during colonoscopy, but may occasionally be indicated during flexible sigmoidoscopy (see Chapter 9). It must be stressed that endoscopic polypectomy should not be taken lightly, and extensive training with a preceptor should be completed before performing polypectomy. Complete bowel preparation is mandatory prior to colonic electrosurgery in order to prevent explosion of combustible gases. Prothrombin time and platelet count should be done to exclude a significant coagulopathy. Aspirin containing compounds may alter platelet function and should not have been taken during the week prior to or after polypectomy.

Principles of Electrosurgery

The endoscopist should be fully competent at diagnostic flexible sigmoidoscopy and well versed in the principles of electrosurgery before attempting endoscopic polypectomy. Papers by Barlow[1] and Curtiss[4] are excellent concise reviews of endoscopic electrosurgery.

High *radio* or frequency current of about 1 million *Hz* is used for endoscopic electrosurgery and is safe because no electrical "shock" or danger to cardiac muscle occurs. By contrast, frequencies below approximately 100,000 *Hz* may produce electrical shock. Two types of electrical current are employed. The *electrocutting* current results in severing of tissue by the thin wire electrode producing an explosion of cells. The depth is shallow and the cutting properties good, but it has poor hemostatic properties. *Electrocoagulation* current results in dessication of tissue. The depth is greater and hemostatic properties are good, but this current has poor cutting properties. Electrosurgical generators utilize both electrocutting and electrocoagulation currents. Some generate a mixed or *blended* current automatically, while others must be pre-set to the desired levels of "cut" and "coag." Both types of current are necessary for adequate polypectomy. The operator should be thoroughly familiar with his or her unit. When a new unit is acquired, it is helpful to check with other operators to find out which settings have worked best. The unit should be checked for proper functioning before each polypectomy and also checked periodically by electrical personnel to insure that the power output remains adequate at each setting.

Current density is an extremely important concept in electrosurgery. It is expressed in amp/cm² and is a measure of intensity. In its simplest form, current density is inversely related to the area through which a given current is passed. The smaller the area, the higher the current density and the greater the heat generated.[1,4] During polypectomy the snare electrode is tightened around the stalk of the polyp, producing a small area for effective electrocoagulation. On the other hand, the large electrode or plate for skin contact causes a barely perceptible heat increase in the skin. Figure 3-25 illustrates that the stalk of a polyp, when snared and tightened, represents a very small cross-sectional area (0.25 cm²).[1] Thus, electrocoagulation of the stalk will produce a high current density and a large temperature rise necessary for adequate polypectomy. The area at the base of the polyp has a larger cross sectional area (1.0 cm²), with a lower current density and thus experiences only a small temperature rise with no or minimal tissue necrosis. The large dermal plate on the patient with an area of 25 cm² has a very small current density, producing only a minute and inapparent temperature rise.

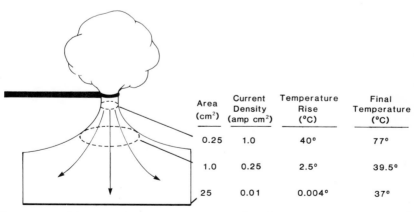

Area (cm²)	Current Density (amp cm²)	Temperature Rise (°C)	Final Temperature (°C)
0.25	1.0	40°	77°
1.0	0.25	2.5°	39.5°
25	0.01	0.004°	37°

Figure 3-25. Temperature rise is proportional to the square of the current density in each cross-sectional area. (Permission courtesy of D. Barlow[1])

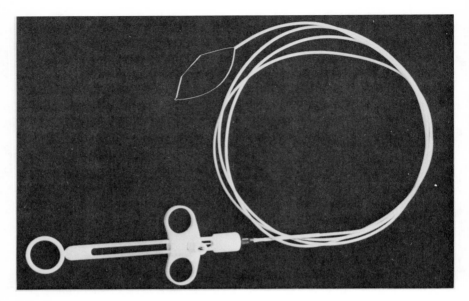

Figure 3-26. Polypectomy snare *(semi-hexagonal shape)* with control handle. Full hexagonal and oval shapes are also available.

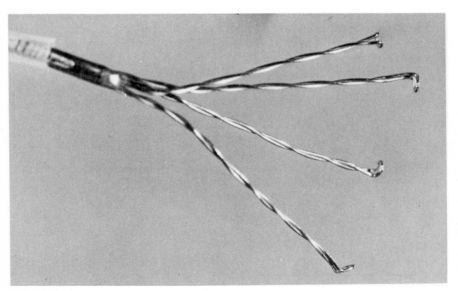

Figure 3-27. Grasping forceps for polyp retrieval. The four grasping tips are blunt ended to avoid colonic injury.

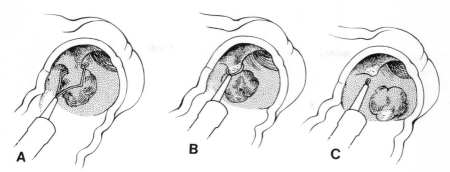

Figure 3-28. Technique for snare cautery of pedunculated polyp. **(A)** Polyp is snared at mid-stalk level. **(B)** Catheter tip pushed to touch stalks; snare loop tightened; electrocautery applied until visible whitening occurs around loop. **(C)** Loop tightened with each burst of current until polyp drops away from stalk.

The snares employed in polypectomy are thin wire electrodes in various shapes controlled by a handle (Fig. 3-26), which also allows for rotation of the snare. Grasping forceps (Fig. 3-27) can be inserted after a polyp has been severed. The polyp may then be grasped and removed, along with the sigmoidoscope. Smaller polyps may be aspirated through the suction channel and collected in a *sputum trap*. Complete reviews of the technique of polypectomy are available.[3,5]

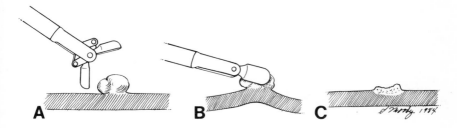

Figure 3-29. Technique of *hot biopsy* for small (5-mm diameter or less) sessile polyps. **(A)** Grasp polyp with insulated forceps. **(B)** Tent polyp away from mucosa, and apply electrocautery for 2–3 seconds. **(C)** Electrocoagulated base.

Technique of Polypectomy[3,5]

Pedunculated polyps   The tip of the instrument is positioned 2-to-3 cm distal to the polyp (Fig. 3-28). The snare is then advanced through the instrument channel and opened under direct vision in the lumen of the colon. The snare is placed over the head of the polyp and maneuvered to the mid-stalk. If the snare is placed too close to the bowel wall, perforation may occur. The sheath of the snare is placed against the stalk and the assistant closes the snare slowly until the head of the polyp becomes congested and blue–red. The head of the polyp should be positioned centrally in the lumen and not in contact with the opposite wall, because application of current can cause a burn on the opposite wall. Electrocoagulation is applied by short bursts of 2–3 seconds each. When the base of the stalk begins to whiten, the snare is tightened further during each burst of current. When the stalk is resected, the snare will perceptively "give," and the polyp will drop away from the bowel wall into the lumen. The polyp can be removed with the grasping forceps or by resnaring. Small polyps can be suctioned into a trap for removal. The polypectomy site should be inspected for completeness of polypectomy and presence of bleeding.

Small sessile polyps (5 mm or less)   Small polyps (Fig. 3-29) may be easily removed with the *hot biopsy* forceps, which are biopsy forceps insulated for electrosurgery. The polyp is grasped and tented away from the wall, and the current is applied for two to three seconds. The polyp can then be pulled away, leaving a coagulated site with destruction of the remainder of the polyp, while the tissue in the biopsy cup remains intact and available for histological review. Sometimes two or three hot biopsies may be needed for complete removal of 4–5 mm polyps.

Medium sized sessile polyps (6 mm to 1.5 cm)   Sessile polyps up to 1.5 cm (Fig. 3-30) can be removed in one stage by snare if a *pseudostalk* is produced. The polyp is grasped with the snare and the base is nar-

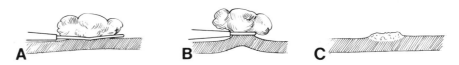

A   B   C

Figure 3-30. Technique for removing medium sized (6–15 mm diameter) sessile polyp. **(A)** Polyp is snared. **(B)** Snare tightened and polyp tented to produce a pseudostalk. **(C)** Electrocoagulated base.

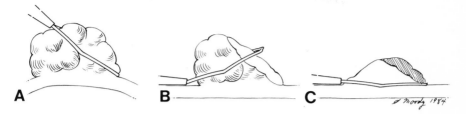

Figure 3-31. Technique for *piecemeal* removal of large sessile polyp (1.5 cm or greater diameter). **(A)** Right portion of polyp snared and resected. **(B)** Left portion of polyp snared and resected. **(C)** Remaining central portion snared and resected.

rowed to 3-5 mm to produce a pseudostalk, which allows current density to be highest at that area. Resection is then accomplished in a manner similar to that of the pedunculated polyp. After resection a wide coagulated base will be seen. The risk of perforation is probably greater after removal of sessile polyps than after removal of pedunculated polyps.

Large sessile polyps (greater than 1.5 cm diameter)   Sessile polyps of from 1.5–8 cm (Fig.3-31) can be successfully removed, but must be done in a "piecemeal" fashion. Depending on the size of the lesion, from two to five pieces are resected until the lesion is removed. Two or more sessions may be necessary. All pieces should be submitted for histopathology, since malignant degeneration is very common in large lesions. The risk of bleeding or perforation is greater with removal of polyps of this size, and this technique should only be undertaken by experienced examiners.

References

1. Barlow DE: Endoscopic applications of electrosurgery: a review of basic principles. Gastrointest Endosc 28:73–76, 1982.
2. Coller JA: Techniques of flexible fiberoptic sigmoidoscopy. Surg Clin N Amer 60:465–479, 1980.
3. Cotton PB, Williams CB: Practical Gastrointestinal Endoscopy (2nd Ed). London, Blackwell Scientific Publication, 1982, pp. 199–235.
4. Curtiss LE: High frequency currents in endoscopy: A review of principles and precautions. Gastrointest Endosc 20:9–12, 1973.
5. Frühmorgen P: Therapeutic colonoscopy, in Hunt RH and Waye JD (Eds.), colonoscopy Techniques. London, Chapman & Hall Ltd., 1981, pp. 199–235.
6. Hocutt JE, Jaffe R, Owens GM, Walters DT: Flexible Fiberoptic Sigmoidoscopy. AFP 26:133–141, 1982.

4

The Procedure Form and Basis
of Informed Consent

THE PROCEDURE FORM

The record of observations and pathologic findings noted during any procedure is an important medical document. The amount of information recorded, both positive and negative, reflects the experience and attention to detail by the examiner. It is important that the medical record be not only accurate but also complete. Too often the only record of a procedure is a sentence or two on the patient's progress sheet, stating that the procedure was simply "negative" or just describing the major pathology. This sketchy and inadequate style of medical record keeping reflects the examiner's lack of understanding of the importance of complete records and may imply a superficially performed procedure.

Two desirable features of a procedure form are that it be concise and clear, and that it be organized in a logical sequence, usually based on anatomy. Some of the specific characteristics of an adequate procedure report include the following:

- Date of procedure
- Patient name, location, and identifying hospital number
- Indication for procedure
- Instrument employed
- Patient position
- Name and dose of premedications
- Type and adequacy of bowel preparation
- Concise statement of both positive and negative findings
- Illustration of findings when appropriate
- Patient tolerance and complications
- Final impression and recommendations
- Name and signature of examiner

The procedure report is often dictated but may also be written on a standard flexible sigmoidoscopy form. At our institution we employ a simple standard medical record form that contains all of the above characteristics that can be easily checked or briefly notated. A standard form can also serve as a reference list for dictation. Our form is a single sheet that contains thirteen items to be completed by the examiner (Fig. 4-1). The form is printed on a three-part, carbonless paper with white, yellow, and pink sheets for distribution to the permanent chart, billing service, and our endoscopy unit files. The date, location of hospital or clinic, hospital number, name, and birthdate of the patient are stamped or written in the upper right corner of the form. The indication for the examination, instrument used, patient position, adequacy of bowel preparation, and medication employed are noted.

The results of external anal inspection are recorded first. Significant findings to be noted include evidence of prior surgery, external hemorrhoids or tags, altered hair distribution, and dermal changes suggesting chronic drainage or irritation. A sentinel tag, usually seen in the posterior midline, is a clue to an anal fissure at its base. Anal fistulae may be manifest by their secondary, external openings. The findings from digital examination are then recorded, paying special attention to anal sphincter tone (increased, normal, or poor), prostate size and consistency, gross or occult blood, and palpable lesions in the presacral hollow, the rectum, or Blummer's shelf (pouch of Douglas).

Even though anoscopy is generally performed at the end of the procedure during slow withdrawal of the flexible instrument, anal findings are recorded first in their anatomical sequence. Anoscopic features that should be noted include internal hemorrhoids, anal fissure or fistulae, stricture, or cryptitis, which is often associated with hypertrophy of the anal papillae. These papillae, as a consequence of chronic inflammation, may enlarge to form one or more elongated anal polyps that are readily palpable and visible on anal examination. These inflammatory polyps are generally white in color, located on the dentate line, and covered with squamous epithelium. In contrast to neoplastic polyps, anal polyps have no malignant potential. Since they have tactile sensitivity, some form of anesthesia is required for removal.

The results of flexible sigmoidoscopy are then recorded and insertion distance or extent of the colonic mucosa visualized is noted. If the examination is limited, the reason (i.e., spasm, stricture, poor preparation, or obstructing lesion) should be noted. The characteristics of the rectal and colonic mucosa that should be routinely noted include color, vascular pattern, and presence or absence of friability and granularity. The colonic mucosa is normally salmon-pink in color with a visible vascular pattern and a glossy sheen on illumination. The absence of a

The Oregon Health Sciences University
Hospital and Clinics

FLEXIBLE SIGMOIDOSCOPY

Date
Location   Bldg.   Fl.   Rm.

Unit No.
Name
Birthdate

1. Indication for Examination:
2. Instrument(s):
3. Position: Inverted   Sims
4. Medication(s):
5. Preparation: Good   Fair   Poor
6. Anal Inspection: Hemorrhoidal tags   Dermal changes
                               Sentinel tag   Fistulae
7. Digital Exam: Sphincter tone   Shelf
                               Prostate   Bleeding
8. Anoscopy: Hemorrhoids   Cryptitis
                               Fissure   Stricture
                               Fistulae   Other
9. Sigmoidoscopy: Distance Cm:
   Mucosa: Sketch polyps or masses
      Color: and note the following:
      Vascular pattern: X = highest point reached
      Friability (0–4+):   # = inflammation
      Granularity (0–4+):   S = snare cautery of polyp
   Valves: Sharp or Blunt   B = biopsy
   Luminal contents: p = photography
   Diverticula:
   Ulceration:
   Polyps:
   Neoplasm:
10. Biopsy Taken:
11. Patient Tolerance:
12. Impression:

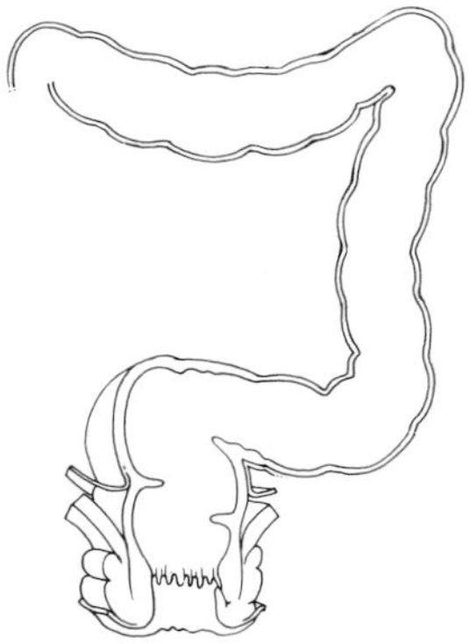

13. Recommendation:

_____ M.D.
Signature/Staff

Figure 4-1. A procedure form for flexible sigmoidoscopy.

vascular pattern suggests mucosal edema. The presence of erythema and edema in the rectum may be due to chemical irritation from enema preparation or to early colitis, particularly when abnormalities persist into the sigmoid colon. Friability denotes increased vascularity from inflammation of the mucosa. The inflamed colonic mucosa undergoes a sequence of progressive changes from no friability (normal), to erythema and petechial changes (nonspecific), to progressive degrees of friability (acute inflammation), to spontaneous friability (severe inflammation). Friability may be arbitrarily graded as 1 + for petechial bleeding, 2–3 + for variable degrees of moderate friability, and 4 + for spontaneous or severe friability. Granularity results from inflammation which transforms the normal smooth and glistening mucosa into an irregular and nodular surface. This also occurs in progressive sequence from a fine granular surface (fine sandpaper), to variable degrees of mucosal nodularity, and finally to a cobblestoned surface with marked mucosal irregularities projecting into the lumen. These granular changes can also be arbitrarily graded in severity—with fine granularity being 1 +, variable moderate granularity 2–3 +, and marked mucosal cobblestoning being 4 +. In general, friability correlates with acute disease activity, whereas granularity without friability denotes chronic inflammatory changes. These findings can be utilized in assessing the degree of acute inflammation and its resolution in patients with colitis.

The rectal valves refer to the three valves of Houston. The left lower valve is located 3–5 cm from the anus, the right middle valve 6–10 cm from the anus, and the left upper valve 8–13 cm from the anus. The valves appear as sharp, crescentic folds projecting into the lumen after insufflation of air. The rectal valves should be observed and noted if they are sharp (i.e., normal) or blunted (i.e., moderate to severe colitis and/or submucosal fibrosis).

Luminal contents refer to the presence of stool, blood, pus, or mucus. These contents can be aspirated into a suction trap at the time of flexible sigmoidoscopy and specimens examined for fecal leukocytes, occult blood, ova and parasites, and bacterial culture and sensitivity.

The presence or absence of pathologic lesions such as diverticula, ulcerations, polyps, and neoplasm are then noted and recorded. The characteristics of these lesions, such as location, size, morphology, and surface mucosa should be carefully described. When a biopsy is taken, it is important to record its location in centimeters from the anus and its source, i.e., from normal mucosa or from a lesion.

Adequacy of patient tolerance and cooperation is recorded as baseline for future examinations. In occasional cases, poor tolerance and/or cooperation signal the need for sedation before repeat examination. Any unusual patient response such as severe pain, distention, hypotension, angina, arrhythmia, vasovagal response, or bleeding, should be noted.

A diagram of the colon allows graphic representation of the various features listed, i.e., maximum distance examined and sites of inflammation, snare polypectomy, biopsy, and/or photographs. Completion of the diagram allows for a quick assessment of what has been written and is of particular value when the record is illegible.

The final impression and recommendations are then summarized from the recorded data on the procedure form.

Our procedure form is a single sheet, simple to complete, thorough in detail and important for longitudinal patient care. We have used this procedure form in our institution for several years with good acceptance by physicians.

THE BASIS OF INFORMED CONSENT

The ultimate goals of informed consent are shared decision making and self determination. Some guidelines[1] for obtaining informed consent for a procedure are listed:

1. The person performing the procedure should obtain the consent.
2. Disclosure requirements should be met:
    - explanation of the nature of the procedure
    - explanation of the purpose of the procedure
    - explanation of the inherent risks and benefits of the procedure
    - explanation of the alternatives to the proposed treatment
    - explanation of the consequences of not having the procedure.
3. Questions regarding the procedure should be solicited and answered.
4. The patient should be informed that he may withdraw from the treatment at any time.
5. A witness should be present when possible.
6. Specific forms should be developed and used.

The individual who is to perform the procedure should obtain the consent. An associate, house officer, or paramedic is not adequate because all the facts, risks, and problems may not be discussed. Personal contact also enhances the rapport and is a significant factor in procedure tolerance and future patient management.

The disclosure requirements are the core of the consent form. They involve discussion of the nature of flexible sigmoidoscopy, such as explanation of instrumentation, air insufflation, biopsy, and/or poly-pectomy procedures. Visual aids may be helpful to demonstrate the procedure. The purpose of the procedure, that is the diagnosis and/or therapy of the presenting problem, should be stated. The major risks and benefits of the procedure and their frequencies should be high-lighted in both verbal and written form. The latter does not require an exhaustive review of every conceivable complication, but the most com-mon risks and their management should be addressed. The alternatives available to evaluate the patient's problem should be explained, includ-ing the possibility of not performing the procedure. It is important to explain to the patient the consequences of *not* having the procedure performed. Record any statement of refusal and the patient's under-standing of the consequences of that decision.

The patient should be given ample time for discussion and ques-tions. Patients are often overwhelmed by the process leading to sigmo-idoscopy and fear the procedure, and thus are reticent to ask questions. Family members should be included in the interview when appropriate. Promoting a give-and-take discussion will help the patient understand the procedure and allay some fears. It is important the patient be informed that he may withdraw from the treatment program at any time without penalty.

It is legally a good idea, if possible, to have a witness present during the interview and not merely when consent is signed. The witness can verify the content of the discussion, the disclosure facts and the ques-tions or concerns of the patient. The ideal witness is a person who is not a member of the operative team. A family member can serve and sign as a witness.

For special procedures such as flexible sigmoidoscopy, it is useful to have a specific consent form. This form should be simple and specif-ically address the procedure in terms of risks and complications. Hos-pital consent forms are usually too general to be of value in this situation. We have used the following short description on our standard hospital form to obtain informed consent:

> The procedure to be performed is a flexible sigmoidoscopy. This procedure may also require intravenous pain medication and sedatives, biopsy or snare polypectomy. The risks of bleeding (less than one in 1000 cases) and tearing a hole (perforation) in the bowel (less than one in 1000 cases), which may require surgery, have been explained and are accepted.

This statement addresses in simple language the two major risks of flexible sigmoidoscopy, their relative frequencies, and the possible need for surgery to manage these complications.

It is important for each examiner to know the standards of disclo-sure for his state or country, since they may vary depending on the jurisdiction. The material presented in this chapter is meant to be only a general guideline. It is recommended that each examiner obtain legal counsel regarding the most appropriate consent form for flexible sigmoidoscopy in his or her practice environment.

REFERENCES

1. Plumeri PA: The gastroenterologist and the doctrine of informed consent. J Clin Gastroenterol 5:185–187, 1983.

5

Comparison of Available Flexible Sigmoidoscopes

MANUFACTURERS AND PURCHASE STRATEGIES

Flexible sigmoidoscopes are produced by five manufacturers and available in two general categories based on their working length: 60-cm (actually 60-cm to 72.5-cm) and 35-cm insertion tube lengths. Each of the five companies produces one or more 60-cm instruments (8 models available), but only three companies are currently making 35-cm sigmoidoscopes (4 models available). One company makes a 30-cm *conversion sleeve* attachment to create a functional 35-cm flexible sigmoidoscope by preventing insertion of 30-cm of the standard 65-cm instrument. The name, address and telephone number of each manufacturer and current 60-cm and 35-cm flexible sigmoidoscopes available by model number are shown in Table 5-1.*

The data reviewed in this chapter should allow the prospective buyer of a new flexible sigmoidoscope to become knowledgeable and conversant with important instrument specifications (e.g., working length, tube diameter, biopsy/suction channel diameter, manual versus automatic air/water feeding) and compare relative purchase prices. The decision to purchase an individual model of flexible sigmoidoscope from a particular manufacturer should be preceded by a review of available specifications and prices as outlined in this chapter and also an assessment of individual need and anticipated usage. The shorter and less expensive flexible sigmoidoscopes are relatively easy to operate

---

*The information provided in this chapter was compiled and updated to September 1984 from correspondence with each manufacturer. More recent information regarding improved or new models should be requested from the central office or local representative of each manufacturer.

Table 5-1

Manufacturers of Flexible Sigmoidoscopes and Available Models
(September 1984)

Manufacturer	Models	
	60-cm	35-cm
Reichert Fiber Optics Division of Warner-Lambert Technologies, Inc. 122 Charlton Street Southbridge, MA 01550 (617) 765–9744	SC-5	FPS-3 SC-35
American ACMI Division of American Hospital Supply Corporation 300 Stillwater Avenue P.O. Box 1971 Stamford, CT 06904 (203) 357–8300 TELEX 99–6466	T-91S TX-91S	None*
Fujinon Inc. 672 White Plains Road Scarsdale, NY 10583 (914) 472–9800 TELEX: SCDL 131642	SIG-E2 SIG-PC	PRO-PC
Olympus Corporation Medical Instrument Division 4 Nevada Drive Lake Success, NY 11042 (516) 488–3880 TELEX: 96–0199 Olympus Lake	OSF CF-P10S	OSF-35
Pentax Precision Instrument Corporation 30 Ramland Road Orangeburg, NY 10962 (914) 365–0700 (800) 431–5880	FS-34A	None

*Conversion sleeve attachment available to create a 35-cm flexible sigmoidoscope from the 65-cm instrument.

and satisfactory for routine diagnostic sigmoidoscopy by generalists (family physicians, internists, and general surgeons). By contrast, the longer and more expensive instruments are generally preferred by specialists (gastroenterologists and colorectal surgeons), who are experienced in colonoscopy and desire complete diagnostic and therapeutic capabilities in a flexible sigmoidoscope. Another important consideration in the purchase of a sigmoidoscope is the availability and service of the local representative of each company. Factors such as prompt communication, provision of literature and/or personal display of instruments, availability of loan equipment, repair time and costs, and overall local reputation should be assessed. Physicians or hospitals already owning upper endoscopes or colonoscopes from one manufacturer will generally want to purchase a flexible sigmoidoscope from the same company, since ancillary equipment (i.e., light sources, teaching attachment, and photographic equipment) will be compatible. Finally, consultation with several colleagues who have extensive experience in flexible sigmoidoscopy regarding overall satisfaction with individual models and instrument companies can provide insights not available from local representatives or literature. The relatively brief time required to obtain the above information is well-spent to insure purchase of the correct flexible sigmoidoscope for one's individual needs.

In the next two sections of this chapter individual specifications and prices of the 60-cm and the 35-cm instruments are compared. This technical data provided from each of the five manufacturers is compiled in tabular form for both the 60-cm and the 35-cm instruments to allow easy comparison of individual features and prices. We do not address the more subjective aspects of these instruments, such as quality of optics and ease of insertion, since we have not directly studied these characteristics and no comparative studies of different models are available. A *Consumer Reports* type of analysis is needed to provide physicians impartial and scientific data comparing the specifications, optical quality, ease of operation, frequency of repair, and costs of flexible sigmoidoscopes to identify the "best buy" of available instruments.

60-CM FLEXIBLE SIGMOIDOSCOPES

Flexible sigmoidoscopes with an insertion tube working length generally between 60 to 65 cm (called the 60-cm flexible sigmoidoscope) are the instruments currently in widespread use by gastroenterologists and colorectal surgeons. Slightly longer prototype instruments (80-100 cm) were briefly used during the early developmental phase of flexible sigmoidoscopy but are no longer available. The specifications and prices

Table 5-2
Specifications and Cost of 60-cm Flexible Sigmoidoscopes

	Reichert	American ACMI	
	SC-5	TX-91S	T-91S
Working length of insertion tube	65 cm	62 cm	65 cm
Outer diameter of insertion tube	13.6 mm	13 mm	13 mm
Channel diameter	3.2 mm	3.3 mm	3.3 mm
Tip deflection	U/D 180° L/R 160°	U/D 180° L/R 180°	U/D 180° L/R 165°
Air feeding	Automatic	Automatic	Automatic
Water feeding	Manual	Automatic or manual	Manual
Suction	Automatic, external	Automatic, internal	Automatic, internal
Field of view	100°	90°	75°
Depth of field	10–70 mm	3–100 mm	3–100 mm
Price	$2650 (light source included)	$4350	$3725

U/D = up-down direction.
L/R = left-right direction.

of the eight currently available 60-cm flexible sigmoidoscopes produced by the five manufacturers are listed in Table 5-2. Reichert Fiber Optics, the first company to introduce a 60-cm instrument in early 1975, makes a relatively inexpensive 65-cm flexible sigmoidoscope, model number SC-5 (Fig. 5-1). This new instrument was made available in 1984 as a replacement of model number SC-4B. American ACMI produces two slightly different and similarly priced 60-cm instruments, the 62-cm TX-91S (Fig. 5-2) and the 65-cm T-91S. A new American ACMI model, the AC-S, with a larger suction channel and improved optics, is scheduled to be available in early 1985. Fujinon Inc. manufactures two 60-cm flexible sigmoidoscopes, the fully automatic long 72.5-cm model number SIG-E2 and the less expensive 65-cm SIG-PC (Fig. 5-3). Olympus

Fujinon		Olympus		Pentax
SIG-E2	SIG-PC	OSF	CF-P10S	FS-34A
72.5 cm	65 cm	60 cm	63 cm	62 cm
13 mm	13 mm	12.2 mm	12.2 mm	11.5 mm
3.7 mm	3.7 mm	3.2 mm	3.2 mm	3.5 mm
U/D 180° L/R 160°	U/D 180° L/R 160°	U/D 180° L/R 160°	U/D 180° L/R 160°	U/D 180° L/R 160°
Automatic	Automatic,	Automatic,	Automatic,	Automatic,
Automatic	Manual	Manual	Automatic or manual	Automatic
Automatic, external & internal	Automatic, external	Automatic, external	Automatic, internal	Automatic, external
105°	105°	100°	120°	95°
2–120 mm	4–120 mm	3–100 mm	5–100 mm	3–100 mm
$4200 ($4500 with light source)	$2700 ($2900 with light source)	$2900	$5400	$3250 ($3500 with light source)

Corporation produces two instruments, the 60-cm model number OSF and the more expensive totally immersible CF-P10S (Fig. 5-4). Pentax makes available a single moderately priced 60-cm instrument, the 62-cm model number FS-34A (Fig. 5-5). The individual specifications are compared in the following sections.

Working Length of Insertion Tube

The working length of the insertion tube refers to the actual length of instrument that can be inserted via the anus into the colon. The most popular working lengths are 62-65 cm, but actual working lengths vary from 60 cm for the Olympus OSF to 72.5 cm for the Fujinon SIG-E2. Some models, such as the Fujinon SIG-E2, have graduated flexibility of

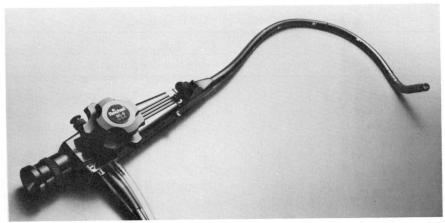

Figure 5-1. 65-cm flexible sigmoidoscope by Reichert Fiber Optics, model SC-5.

the insertion tube with the proximal portion near the control head more rigid and the distal portion more flexible.

Outer Diameter of Insertion Tube

The outer diameter of the insertion tube varies over a narrow range from 11.5 mm for the Pentax FS-34A, the slimmest model, to 13.6 mm

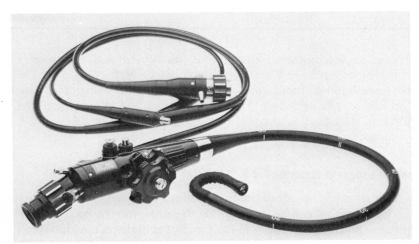

Figure 5-2. 62-cm flexible sigmoidoscope by American ACMI, model TX-91S

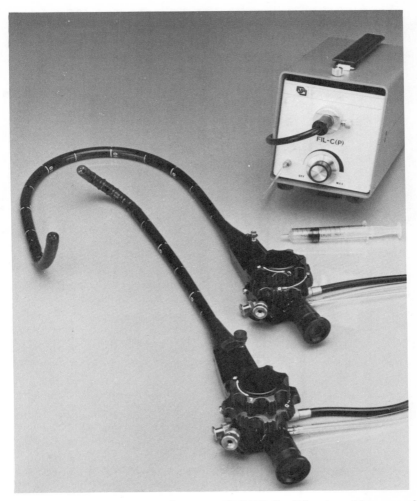

Figure 5-3. 65-cm SIG-PC and 35-cm PRO-PC flexible sigmoidoscopes by Fujinon, Inc.

for the Reichert SC-5, the largest diameter. The other six models vary in outer diameter from 12.2 mm to 13 mm. In spite of claims that instruments with a smaller outer diameter are inserted with less patient discomfort, this contention has not been proven by comparative studies. However, the smaller outer diameter instruments will allow easier passage through rectosigmoid strictures resulting from scarring, diverticular disease, or neoplasms.

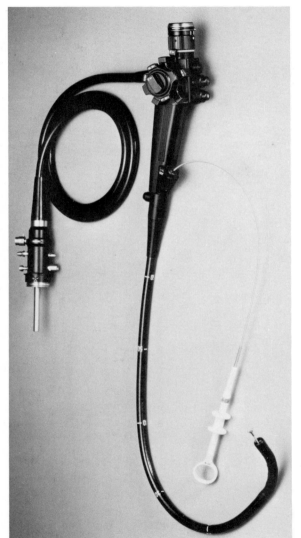

Figure 5-4. 60-cm flexible sigmoidoscope by Olympus Corporation, model CF-P10S.

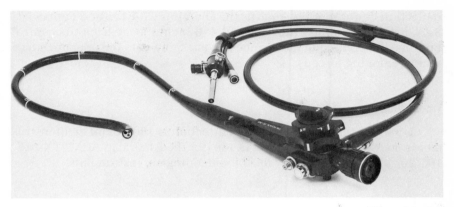

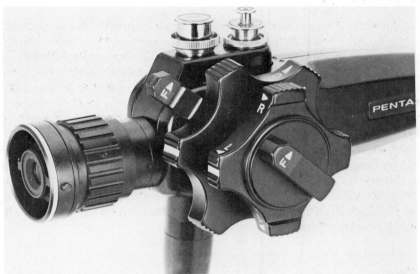

Figure 5-5. 62-cm flexible sigmoidoscope by Pentax, model FS-34A. (A) Instrument and umbulical cord. (B) Control head.

Channel Diameter

Channel diameters vary from 3.2 mm for the Reichert SC-5 and both Olympus models to 3.7 mm for the Fujinon SIG-E2 and SIG-PC. The larger channel sizes improve suction capability, an important consideration in poorly-prepared colons with retained liquid material. The larger channels also allow usage of bigger biopsy instruments and other accessories and permit easier passage of this equipment with full tip deflection. Some models, such as the Olympus CF-P10S and Pentax FS-34A, have the channel inlet located 4–6 inches away from the control buttons, thus reducing the chance of back spray onto the operator's face when removing forceps.

Tip Deflection

Tip deflection in the up–down direction is 180° for all eight instruments. Left–right tip deflection is 180° for the American ACMI TX-91S, 165° for the T-91S and 160° for the remaining six instruments.

Air and Water Feeding

All eight instruments permit automatic air insufflation via a button on the control head. By contrast, water feeding may be achieved in the various models either manually by syringe injection, automatically by a control button, or both automatically and manually. Automatic water feeding, which delivers a low velocity stream of water to the distal surface of the endoscope, is convenient and routinely used for cleaning a soiled lens surface during examination. More forcible manual injection of water is occasionally necessary to dislodge particles of stool trapped in the distal lens hood and not removable by passage of a catheter or forceps through the biopsy channel. The American ACMI TX-91S and the Olympus CF-P10S are the only models that have a separate back-up port on the control head for auxillary manual syringe injection of water. The Reichert SC-5 has a unique forward irrigation jet for washing and biopsy site preparation.

Suction

Suction is also automatic in all eight instruments and activated by a button on the control head of the instrument. The individual models vary in the way tubing from a suction source is connected to the instrument suction channel at the control head. In some models the tubing from a suction pump is external to the umbilical cord and attaches separately at the control head, while in other models the tubing is built into the umbilical cord. An external attachment of suction tubing has the advantage of quick separation from the control head of the instrument for aspiration or flushing when it becomes clogged during an examination. The Fujinon SIG-E2 is the only model that can be operated with internal suction, external suction, or both together.

Angle and Depth of Viewing Field

The field of view, or angle of viewing field, varies from 90° to 105° for six models, while the American ACMI T-91S has a relatively narrow angle of 75° and the Olympus CF-P10S a relatively wide angle of 120°. The depth of field for the Reichert SC-5 is limited to 10–70 mm, but the other seven models range 2–5 mm to 100–120 mm. These optical specifications, along with the engineering of fiberoptic bundles and lens systems, are important determinants of the overall optical quality of the various instruments. The wider fields and greater depths of view reduce blind spots and may make insertion of the instrument easier by identifying the luminal direction around sharp sigmoid colon angulations.

Price

Prices for the various models, as of September 1984, are shown in Table 5-2. The least expensive model is the Reichert SC-4B at $2650, which includes the light source. However, this model also has the largest outer diameter, a relatively small channel diameter, a limited angle and depth of viewing field, and manual water feeding. At $5100 the most expensive model is the Olympus CF-P10S, which is totally immersible without damage to the control body, has a relatively small outer diameter , is fully automatic, and has the widest field of view. The other models are priced between these extremes. In the middle price range, the fully automatic American ACMI TX-91S, Fujinon SIG-E2 and Pentax FS-34A are more expensive than the American ACMI T-91S and Fujinon SIG-PC with manual water feeding. Other factors, such as external versus internal suction capability and field of view, should also be considered in this price range. In the absence of direct unbiased comparative studies of these eight models, the prospective buyer must compare price with specifications and make use of purchase strategies outlined in the first part of this chapter. The companies or their local representatives will sometimes put together flexible sigmoidoscope packages including such accessories as light sources, biopsy equipment, cameras, etc. at substantial savings.

35-CM FLEXIBLE SIGMOIDOSCOPES

Flexible sigmoidoscopes with an insertion tube working length of 35 cm were made available only a few years ago. The usefulness of a flexible sigmoidoscope of this length is still undergoing study; however, its ease of insertion, good patient acceptance, and reasonable yield of

Table 5-3
Specifications and Cost of 35-cm Flexible Sigmoidoscopes

	Reichert		Fujinon	Olympus
	FPS-3	SC-35	PRO-PC	OSF-35
Working length of insertion tube	35 cm	35 cm	35 cm	35 cm
Outer diameter of insertion tube	13.2 mm	13.4 mm	13 mm	12.2 mm
Channel diameter	2.6 mm	2.6 mm	3.7 mm	3.2 mm
Tip deflection	U/D 175° L/R 0°	U/D 170° L/R 140°	U/D 180° L/R 160°	U/D 180° L/R 160°
Air feeding	Manual	Automatic	Automatic	Automatic
Water feeding	Manual	Manual	Manual	Manual
Suction	Automatic, external	Automatic, external	Automatic, external	Automatic, external
Field of view	75°	90°	105°	100°
Depth of field	10–70 mm	10–70 mm	4–120 mm	3–100 mm
Price	$1475 (light source included)	$2150 (light source included)	$2500 ($2700 with light source)	$2700

U/D = up-down direction.   L/R = left-right direction.

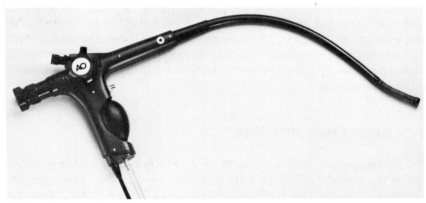

Figure 5-6. 35-cm flexible sigmoidoscope by Reichert Fiber Optics, model FPS-3

polyps and cancer (see Chapter 7), combined with moderate purchase price make this instrument practical for routine diagnostic sigmoidoscopy by physicians in general practice. Four 35-cm flexible sigmoidoscopes are currently produced by three manufacturers (Table 5-3). Reichert Fiber Optics, the first company to produce the 35-cm flexible sigmoidoscope intended for general use in office screening sigmoidoscopy, makes the inexpensive model FPS-3 (Fig.5-6) and also the SC-35. Fujinon Inc. produces one instrument, model number PRO-PC (Fig. 5-3), and the Olympus Corporation manufactures a shorter 35-cm version of their 60-cm OSF called OSF-35.

American ACMI and Pentax do not produce a 35-cm flexible sigmoidoscope. American ACMI, however, offers a unique approach to 35-cm sigmoidoscopy by making a *conversion sleeve*, which attaches to each of their 60-cm instruments (TX-91S and T-91S) and shortens the working length of the insertion tube by 30 cm. This rigid conversion sleeve (model number S3565) attaches to the instrument before examination, shortens the 62–65 cm insertion tube usable length to 32–35 cm, and cannot be removed during the procedure. The sleeve may be used on a regular basis for 35-cm examinations or only during initial flexible sigmoidoscopies (analogous to training wheels on a bicycle) until the examiner feels experienced enough to perform 60-cm flexible sigmoidoscopy. This unique accessory is provided free with purchase of each of the American ACMI 60-cm instruments.

The individual specifications and purchase prices of the four 35-cm flexible sigmoidoscopes are compared in Table 5-3 and discussed briefly below.

Working Length of Insertion Tube

All four models have a 35-cm insertion tube working length.

Outer Diameter of Insertion Tube

The Reichert instruments have the larger outer diameter of 13.2 mm (FPS-3) and 13.4 mm (SC-35), while the Olympus OSF-35 has the smallest diameter of 12.2 mm.

Channel Diameter

The channel size for instrumentation and suction are 2.6 mm in the Reichert FPS-3 and SC-35, 3.2 mm in the Olympus OSF-35, and 3.7 mm in the Fujinon PRO-PC.

Tip Deflection

The Reichert FPS-3 is the only flexible sigmoidoscope with two-way tip deflection ($\pm$ 175° in up–down direction), while the other three models have the more standard four-way tip deflection.

Air and Water Feeding

Air insufflation is controlled automatically by buttons on the control head of all three models except the Reichert FPS-3, which has manual air feeding via an insufflation bulb. Water feeding is manual via syringe for all four models.

Suction

Suction is automatic with the tubing from the suction pump attached externally to the control head of all four instruments.

Angle and Depth of Viewing Field

The variable angle and depth of viewing fields of each of the four models is shown in Table 5-3. The Fujinon PRO-PC and Olympus OSF-35 are nearly comparable and have somewhat wider ranges than the Reichert models.

Price

Reichert manufactures the least expensive 35-cm flexible sigmoidoscopes available. The FPS-3 has a total purchase price of only $1475 with light source included. The major differences in specifications, most notably the two-way tip deflection, manual air feeding and 75° field of view, need to be balanced against this low purchase price. The other three instruments are comparable in price and specifications, except that the Fujinon PRO-PC and Olympus OSF-35 have slightly greater tip deflection capabilities and wider fields of view.

ANCILLARY EQUIPMENT

A large selection of ancillary equipment is available from each of the manufacturers. Many of the accessories, such as light sources, cameras, and teaching attachments, are only compatible with flexible sigmoidoscopes manufactured by the same company. However, most companies also produce adapters that allow use of ancillary equipment with sigmoidoscopes made by another company.

Light Sources

Light sources vary widely in price depending upon their illumination power and source and their photographic capabilities. For example, the basic 150 W halogen Pentax light source (LH-150P) and the similar Olympus light source (CLK-3) list for $595 and $470, respectively. However, the models with automatic photography capability from each of these companies (Pentax LH-150FP and Olympus CLE-4U) triples in price and lists for $1650 and $1660, respectively. Finally, 300 W xenon light sources with automatic, Polaroid, cine, and video photographic capabilities list for approximately $5000. Most companies significantly reduce the cost of the light source if purchased as a package with a flexible sigmoidoscope. For example, the Pentax LH-150P lists for $595 but costs only $250 when purchased as a complete package with FS-34A flexible sigmoidoscope.

Teaching Attachments

Many operators of flexible sigmoidoscopes regularly use a teaching attachment to allow the endoscopy assistant visualization of the colon as he or she advances and torques the instrument and demonstrates pathology to interested observers. These important accessories are not inexpensive, e.g., Reichert TA-1 or TA-2 at $1700, Olympus LS-R at $2295 and LS-10 at $2350, and Pentax FO-T1 at $2350. Most companies make adapters to make sigmoidoscopes and teaching attachments from different companies compatible with one another.

Photographic Equipment

The most popular photographic technique for documentation of sigmoidoscopic findings is to use 35-mm transparency film in a single lens reflex camera attached to a flexible sigmoidoscope that has the capability for automatic photography. All flexible sigmoidoscopes can be used for photography of colonic findings, but some instruments require special adapters while others are designed for easy camera attachment. In addition, some flexible sigmoidoscopes are internally wired for automatic photography when an appropriate light source is used, while other models require manual adjustment of camera settings for each picture. Photographic documentation may also be achieved using 16-mm transparency and 110-mm cartridge film, instant Polaroid, 8 and 16-mm cine and video. The latter special photographic techniques require powerful and expensive xenon light sources. In summary, many variables determine successful photography for individual needs, and the operating manual should be consulted regarding photographic capability, preferred light source, camera and camera adapters, usable type of film, and camera settings.

Electrosurgical Equipment

Most models of 60-cm flexible sigmoidoscopes are engineered with internal wiring for electrical grounding through the light source and thus are safe to use for electrosurgical procedures such as hot biopsy and snare-cautery polypectomy. Other flexible sigmoidoscopes, including all the 35-cm models, are designed primarily for diagnostic purposes and though not internally wired, can be grounded by an external attachment. The instructions in the operating manual of the flexible sigmoidoscope and the cautery unit should be studied and followed carefully when electrosurgery is performed.

Miscellaneous

Other accessories in common use include biopsy forceps, cleaning and cytology brushes, grasping forceps, diathermy snares, and miscellaneous adapters. Prices of these individual items vary but many add several hundred or more dollars to the total package purchase price.

6

Comparison of 60-cm Flexible Sigmoidoscopy
with Rigid Sigmoidoscopy

In 1977 our group reported the first clinical study comparing 60-cm flexible sigmoidoscopy with standard rigid sigmoidoscopy.[2] We studied 120 consecutive patients who were referred for sigmoidoscopy for miscellaneous indications and had agreed to undergo both procedures. Our findings indicated that 60-cm flexible sigmoidoscopy was more valuable than rigid sigmoidoscopy in the detection of colorectal neoplasia, diverticular disease, and inflammatory bowel disease. In addition, no sedation was needed, adequate bowel preparation was easily achieved with one enema, and the procedure time was only a few minutes longer for the flexible examination. Over the next few years, several additional studies comparing both procedures were published. The results of these studies will be outlined and analyzed in this chapter. In addition, the several studies addressing the exact anatomic extent of colon reached during 60-cm flexible sigmoidoscopy will be reviewed.

RESULTS OF STUDIES COMPARING 60-CM FLEXIBLE SIGMOIDOSCOPY WITH RIGID SIGMOIDOSCOPY

Bowel Preparation

Of 10 studies (Table 6-1) specifying the type of bowel preparation and results, half of the investigators employed one enema and the remainder used two enemas. Most authors preferred use of Phospho-Soda enemas, although tap water and saline enemas were also used. The enema preparation used in the comparative sigmoidoscopy studies proved adequate in most cases, with a success rate ranging from 80–98%. It appears that a single enema provides as thorough a bowel

Table 6-1
Bowel Preparation for 60-cm Flexible Sigmoidoscopy

Author*	Patients	Enemas	Enema Type	Inadequate Preparation (%)
Bohlman[2]	120	1	Phospho-Soda	10
Holt[4]	116	1	Phospho-Soda	3
Crespi[3]	488	1	Tap Water[†]	2
Vellacott[19]	350	1	Phospho-Soda	5
Manier[8]	192	1	Phospho-Soda	7
Marks[9]	1012	2	Saline	3
Winnan[20]	342	2	Phospho-Soda	20
Leicester[6]	516	2	Phospho-Soda	21
Meyer[10]	408	2	Phospho-Soda	5
Traul[16]	5000	2	Phospho-Soda	2

*First author and reference number.
†Supplemented by 2 Dulcolax tablets given the day before.

preparation as two enemas. The standard preparation may occasionally need to be augmented in constipated elderly patients by the addition of a laxative the day before the examination.

Insertion Distance

The average insertion distance (Table 6-2) in the comparative sigmoidoscopy studies for the rigid instrument was 20-cm versus 52-cm for the flexible instrument. The true anatomic extent of 60-cm flexible sigmoidoscopy as documented by several investigators will be discussed later in this chapter.

Duration of Examination

The mean time required to perform rigid sigmoidoscopy (Table 6-3) is between 5 and 6 minutes, while the flexible examination takes 8–12 minutes. This difference in time not only reflects the extra length of colon examined by flexible sigmoidoscopy but also includes the additional time required for colonic biopsies and endoscopic photography.

Table 6-2
Insertion Distance During 60-cm Flexible and Rigid Sigmoidoscopy

		Mean Distance (cm)	
Author*	Patients	Flexible	Rigid
Bohlman[2]	120	55	20
Marks[9]	1012	50	20
Winnan[20]	342	50	20
Leicester[6]	516	51	18
Totals	1990	52	20

*First author and reference number.

Another important factor not considered in these studies is the time needed to adequately clean and disinfect flexible instruments between examinations. Since many diagnostic units employ disposable rigid instruments, there is virtually no waiting time between rigid sigmoidoscopy procedures. On the other hand, effective cleaning and disinfection of flexible instruments requires a minimum of 10 minutes. This additional time factor may assume major importance if only a single flexible instrument is available and several cases are scheduled for a single setting.

Table 6-3
Mean Time of Examination

		Mean Time (minutes)	
Author*	Patients	Flexible	Rigid
Bohlman[2]	120	9	6
Marks[9]	1012	6	5
Winnan[20]	342	12	6
Vellacott[19]	350	8	NS[†]
Leicester[6]	516	8	NS
Totals	2340	9	6

*First author and reference number.
†NS = not stated.

Patient Preference and Position of Patient During Examination

Seven comparative studies of 60-cm flexible versus rigid sigmoidoscopy evaluated patient tolerance and preference for one or the other examination. Wide variation in results were noted and are shown in Table 6-4. One study showed a strong patient preference for the flexible exam,[11] and three studies noted a slight patient preference for the flexible exam.[2,8,13] Two studies found patient tolerance and preference essentially the same for both procedures,[17,20] and one study found a moderate patient preference for the rigid examination.[6] Poor procedure tolerance was noted with both examinations in several studies in patients with diverticular disease, colonic spasm, strictures, and prior abdominal surgery.[2,6,9,16]

The patient position was variable for both rigid and flexible sigmoidoscopy. Three groups placed patients in the left lateral (Sims) position while two groups examined patients with both procedures in the inverted position on a sigmoidoscopy table. One group used the inverted position for rigid sigmoidoscopy and left lateral position for flexible sigmoidoscopy. No study directly compared patient or operator preference for left lateral versus inverted position for flexible sigmoidoscopy. Some operators prefer to perform flexible sigmoidoscopy with the patient in the inverted position, as has been traditionally used for rigid sigmoidoscopy, while others prefer the left lateral position as is employed for colonoscopy.

Polyps and Cancers

Six studies summarized in Table 6-5 show a consistent pattern of a larger number of polyps and cancer found during 60-cm flexible sigmoidoscopy than during the rigid procedure. The overall diagnostic yield by flexible sigmoidoscopy compared with rigid sigmoidoscopy is 3.1 fold greater for polyps and 3.5 fold greater for cancer in the six studies. The individual studies showed considerable variation in the comparative yield for polyps and cancer by both procedures (Table 6-5).

It is postulated that approximately 65–70% of polyps throughout the entire colon are within reach of the 60-cm flexible sigmoidoscope.[14] If one-third of these lesions are routinely discovered with the rigid instrument, then approximately 20–25% of the total colonic polyps will be found if only rigid sigmoidoscopy is employed. The concept of screening for colorectal neoplasia and the potential advantages of the flexible instruments is discussed in Chapter 10.

Table 6-4
Patient Preference for Rigid Versus Flexible Sigmoidoscopy

Author*	Patients	Prefer Rigid (%)	Prefer Flexible (%)	No Preference (%)
O'Connor[11]	109	2	94	4
Ribet[13]	125	25	40	35
Manier[8]	192	37	45	18
Bohlman[2]	120	33	43	24
Winawer[17]	108	**	**	—
Winnan[20]	342	**	**	—
Leicester[6]	516	38	—	62

*First author and reference number.
**Equal preference for flexible or rigid sigmoidoscopy.

Diverticular Disease

Colonic diverticula are not found in the rectum and only rarely in the distal sigmoid colon. It is evident from the data in Table 6-6 that only 2% (4 of 235) of patients with diverticular disease were discovered

Table 6-5
Number of Polyps and Cancers Found by Rigid Versus
Flexible Sigmoidoscopy

Author*	Patients (No.)	Polyps Flexible/Rigid	Cancers Flexible/Rigid
Winawer[17]	108	35/3	5/1
Winnan[20]	342	36/6	3/1
Bohlman[2]	120	30/6	6/2
Vellacott[19]	350	45/10	17/2
Leicester[6]	516	64/20	9/2
Marks[9]	1012	253/106	26/11
Totals	2448	463/151 (3.1:1)	66/19 (3.5:1)

*First author and reference number.

Table 6-6
Diagnosis of Diverticulosis and Inflammatory Bowel Disease by Rigid Versus
Flexible Sigmoidoscopy

		Diverticulosis	IBD[+]
Author*	Patients (No.)	Flexible/Rigid	Flexible/Rigid
Winawer[17]	108	13/1	—
Marks[9]	1012	117/1	39/22
Leicester[6]	516	68/2	35/29
Bohlman[2]	120	8/0	9/7
Vellacott[19]	350	29/0	12/10
Totals	2106	235/4 (2%)	95/68 (72%)

*First author and reference number.
[+]Inflammatory Bowel Disease.

during rigid sigmoidoscopy when compared with flexible sigmoidoscopy. The differentiation of complicated diverticular disease from colon carcinoma, Crohn's disease, and ischemic colitis can be difficult by clinical evaluation and barium studies alone. In addition, the thickened and convoluted bowel contour in advanced diverticular disease may obscure polypoid lesions even when double-contrast barium enema examination is performed. Thus, rigid examination has very limited value in studying patients to document evidence of diverticular disease and exclude coexistent disease such as polyps or cancer.

Colitis

Rigid sigmoidoscopy was diagnostic in only 72% (68 of 95 patients) with various types of colitis (Table 6-6). This occurs because of the lack of rectal involvement in a variable number of patients with Crohn's disease, ischemic colitis, antibiotic-associated colitis, and other types of inflammatory bowel disease. The rigid examination is often preferred for initial diagnosis, or monitoring proctitis, and for obtaining deep rectal biopsies. However, the flexible examination can provide further information by determining the extent of colonic involvement or by establishing a diagnosis in diseases that spare the rectum.

Summary of Studies Comparing 60-Cm Flexible with Rigid Sigmoidoscopy

Table 6-7 is a general summary of the similarities and differences between 60-cm flexible sigmoidoscopy and standard 25-cm rigid sigmoidoscopy as reported in the literature.

Table 6-7

Summary of Studies Comparing Flexible (60-cm) with
Rigid (25-cm) Sigmoidoscopy

	Sigmoidoscopy	
	Rigid (25-cm)	Flexible (60-cm)
Sedation	None	None
Preparation	1 or 2 enemas	1 or 2 enemas
Duration	5–6 min	8–12 min
Insertion depth	17–20 cm	50–55 cm
Tolerance	Fair	Usually good
Polyps		3-fold higher yield
Carcinoma		3-fold higher yield
Diverticular disease	Rarely seen	Left-sided seen well
Colitis	Submucosal biopsy; rectal disease	Mucosal biopsy; disease above rectum
Cost of instrument	$300–400	$2650–5000
Cost of procedure (Professional fee)	$35–45	$75–125

ANATOMIC EXTENT OF COLON VISUALIZED DURING 60-CM FLEXIBLE FIBEROPTIC SIGMOIDOSCOPY

A study by Madigan and Halls[7] has shown that the rigid sigmoidoscope, even during full insertion, often pushes the mucosa ahead of the
instrument, limiting the anatomic extent of examination to the rectum
or distal sigmoid colon.

Although the centimeter marks on the flexible fiberoptic sigmoidoscope serve as a rough guide to the length of colon inspected, considerable variation exists in the true anatomic extent of colon examined.
The instrument may form a loop during advancement, and further insertion of the instrument shaft (by more centimeters) may simply distend
distal sigmoid loops without advancing the tip. Insertion of the full 60
cm of the sigmoidoscope may advance the tip to the mid-sigmoid colon
or all the way to the transverse colon. Endoscopic inspection of the
lumen is a poor indicator of the maximal anatomic extent reached.

Table 6-8
Anatomic Extent of Fiberoptic Sigmoidoscopy

Author*	Patients (No.)	Method of Localization	Full 60-cm Insertion (%)	Instrument Tip at or Above Sigmoid-Descending Colon Junction (%)
Ott[12]	42	Plain film + BE[+]	74	94
Bohlman[2]	19	Fluoroscopy + plain film	100	84
Leicester[6]	516	NS[+]	NS	82
Lehman[5]	113	Mucosal clip + BE	55	81
Auslander[1]	NS	Plain film or fluoroscopy	100	75
Theuerkeuf[15]	50	NS	100	69

*First author and reference number.
[+]BE = Barium enema examination.
[+]NS = not stated.

Table 6-9
Insertion Distance During 60-cm Flexible Sigmoidoscopy Versus Anatomic Extent of Colon Visualized

Insertion Distance (cm)	Proximal Extent of Colon Visualized				
	Distal Sigmoid Colon (%)	Sigmoid-Descending Colon Junction (%)	Descending Colon (%)	Splenic Flexure Colon (%)	Transverse Colon (%)
60	100	69–94	23–34	22	7–10
40–59	83–93	27–68	0–20	0–6	0
25–39	0–60	0–13	0	0	0
<25	0	0	0	0	0

Based on studies by Lehman et al.[5] and Ott et al.[12]

Several studies [1,2,5,6,12,15] have used fluoroscopy, plain film of the abdomen, barium enema, and mucosal clipping devices to provide objective data of proximal extent reached by the tip of the flexible sigmoidoscope during examination (Table 6-8). In these studies the examiners achieved full 60-cm insertion in 55–100% of patients. With this reasonably complete insertion of the flexible sigmoidoscope, the sigmoid-descending colon junction was reached in 69–94% of patients. This data suggests that a complete 60-cm flexible sigmoidoscopy has approximately an 80% chance of reaching the sigmoid-descending colon junction and becoming a true *pansigmoidoscopy*. Auslander et al.[1] noted that the physician's estimate of depth of insertion was correct in only 54% of cases and that the insertion distance was underestimated in 8% and overestimated in 38% of cases.

While full 60-cm insertion of the flexible sigmoidoscope often reaches the sigmoid-descending colon (69–94%), there is a marked decrease in anatomic extent of colon visualized when insertion is less than 60-cm (Table 6-9). At the 40–59 cm range of insertion, complete sigmoid visualization is achieved in only 27–68% of the patients. Moreover, with insertion to between 25–39 cm, full sigmoid colon inspection occurs in 0–13% of the patients. This latter figure should be kept in mind when the relative merits of 60-cm versus 35-cm flexible sigmoidoscopy are discussed in Chapter 7.

The 60-cm flexible examination in most reported studies has been performed by accomplished endoscopists, usually gastroenterologists or colorectal surgeons. Questions have been raised[18] regarding whether the nonendoscopist can be taught to use the 60-cm instrument safely and accurately or whether a 35-cm flexible instrument might be preferable. These issues will be discussed in the next chapter.

REFERENCES

1. Auslander MO, Schapiro M: The true depth of insertion of the 60 cm. flexible fiberoptic sigmoidoscope. Gastrointest Endosc (Abstract) 29:192, 1983.
2. Bohlman TW, Katon RM, Lipshutz GR, et al.: Fiberoptic pansigmoidoscopy, an evaluation and comparison with rigid sigmoidoscopy. Gastroenterology 72:644–649, 1977.
3. Crespi M, Casale V, Grassi A: Flexible sigmoidoscopy, a potential advance in cancer control. Gastrointest Endosc 24:291–292, 1978.
4. Holt RW, Wherry DC: Flexible fiberoptic sigmoidoscopy in a surgeon's office. Am J Surg 39:708–710, 1980.
5. Lehman GA, Buchner DM, Lappas JC: Anatomical extent of fiberoptic sigmoidoscopy. Gastroenterology 84:803–808, 1983.
6. Leicester RJ, Hawley RR, Pollett WG, Nichols RJ: Flexible fiberoptic sigmoidoscopy as an outpatient procedure. Lancet 1:34–35, 1982.

7. Madigan MR, Halls JM: The extent of sigmoidoscopy shown on radiographs with reference to the rectosigmoid junction. Gut 9:355–362, 1968.
8. Manier JW: Fiberoptic pansigmoidoscopy: an evaluation of its use in an office practice. Gastrointest Endosc 24:119–120, 1978.
9. Marks G, Boggs W, Castro AF, et al.: Sigmoidoscopic examination with rigid and flexible fiberoptic sigmoidoscopes in the surgeon's office: A comparative prospective study of effectiveness in 1,012 cases. Dis Colon Rectum 22:162–168, 1979.
10. Meyer C, McBride W, Goldblatt RS, et al.: Clinical experience with flexible sigmoidoscopy in asymptomatic and symptomatic patients. Yale J of Biol Med 53:345–352, 1980.
11. O'Connor JJ: Flexible sigmoidoscopy: Is it of value? Am Surg 45:647–648, 1979.
12. Ott DJ, Wu WC, Gelfand DW: Extent of colonic visualization with the fiberoptic sigmoidoscope. J Clin Gastroent 4:337–341, 1982.
13. Ribet A, Escourrou J, Frexinos J, Delpu J: Screening for colorectal tumors. Results of two years experience. Cancer Detection and Prevention 3:449–461, 1980.
14. Tedesco FJ, Waye JD, Avella JR, Villalobas MM: Diagnostic implications of the spatial distribution of colonic mass lesions (polyps and cancers). Gastrointest Endosc 26:95–97, 1980.
15. Theuerkeuf FJ: Rectal and colonic polyp relationships via colonoscopy and fiber sigmoidoscopy. Dis Colon Rectum 21:2–7, 1978.
16. Traul DG, Davis C, Pollack J, Scudamore H: Flexible fiberoptic sigmoidoscopy—the Monroe Clinic experience. Dis Colon Rectum 26:161–166, 1983.
17. Winawer SJ, Leidner SD, Boyle C, Kurtz RC: Comparison of flexible sigmoidoscopy with other diagnostic techniques in the diagnosis of rectocolon neoplasia. Dig Dis Sci 24:277–281, 1979.
18. Winawer SJ, Cummins R, Baldwin MP, Ptak A: A new flexible sigmoidoscope for the generalist. Gastrointest Endosc 28:233–236, 1982.
19. Vellacott KD, Hardcastle JD: An evaluation of flexible fibreoptic sigmoidoscopy. Brit Med J 283:1583–1586, 1981.
20. Winnan G, Berci G, Panish J, et al.: Superiority of the flexible to the rigid sigmoidoscope in routine proctosigmoidoscopy. N Engl J Med 302:1011–1012, 1980.

7

The 60-cm versus the 35-cm Flexible
Sigmoidoscope—The Long and the Short of It

Despite the clear superiority of 60-cm flexible sigmoidoscopy over rigid sigmoidoscopy (see Chapter 6), several authors were skeptical regarding the value of flexible sigmoidoscopy. Schapiro suggested that flexible sigmoidoscopy might be akin to a "half-a-loaf" concept.[10] He expresses concern that the time-honored indications for full colonoscopy might be abandoned in favor of the shorter 60-cm examination. The results of Tedesco et al.[12] would appear to support this concern. He studied the spatial distribution of colonic adenomas and carcinomas during colonoscopy and found that 34% of polyps and 36% of cancers were beyond the 60-cm level. He cautioned that such proximal lesions would be missed by 60-cm flexible sigmoidoscopy.

The fact that a significant percent of lesions occur proximal to 60-cm is indisputable. However, flexible sigmoidoscopy should be viewed in most cases as a replacement for rigid sigmoidoscopy rather than being compared with full colonoscopy. In fact, at our institution, we suspect that one of the major reasons why more colonoscopies are being performed is the increased amount of pathology found by flexible sigmoidoscopy. We heartily agree with the statement, "Flexible sigmoidoscopy is a rich man's version of rigid sigmoidoscopy; it is not a poor man's version of colonoscopy."[14]

Paradoxically, while there is concern over the potential of missed proximal lesions using the 60-cm flexible sigmoidoscope, there is simultaneous enthusiasm by some authors for the use of a shorter flexible 35-cm sigmoidoscope.[5,13,15] It is argued that the 60-cm instrument is not easily mastered by the nonendoscopist and that he may experience a greater frequency of major complications. Studies reporting clinical experience with the shorter flexible sigmoidoscope and evaluating 35-

cm flexible sigmoidoscopy in comparison with 60-cm flexible or rigid sigmoidoscopy will be reviewed in this chapter.

CLINICAL EXPERIENCE WITH THE SHORTER (35-CM) FLEXIBLE SIGMOIDOSCOPE

Sarles et al.[9] studied 165 patients who underwent flexible sigmoidoscopy with a 35-cm instrument by staff gastroenterologists and fellows. They found a mean insertion distance of 29 cm, only mild patient discomfort, and a mean procedure time of only 4.2 minutes. The instrument employed in their study was a low-priced model ($1300, including light source) with two-directional tip control. The authors computed that instrument cost, based on the manufacturer's estimated endoscope life of 800 procedures, was only $1.60 per procedure.

COMPARISON OF 35-CM FLEXIBLE SIGMOIDOSCOPY WITH RIGID SIGMOIDOSCOPY

Grobe et al.[3] studied 71 symptomatic patients with both the rigid 25-cm sigmoidoscope and a 35-cm flexible sigmoidoscope with two-directional tip control. The results of this small series by experienced endoscopists are impressive (Table 7-1). The 35-cm flexible examination required about the same procedure time as rigid sigmoidoscopy, visualized 8.5 cm more of bowel, and was associated with much less discomfort. In addition, of 16 adenomatous polyps detected during the

Table 7-1
Results of 35-cm Flexible Versus Rigid Sigmoidoscopy*

	Sigmoidoscopy	
	Flexible (35-cm)	Rigid (25-cm)
Examination time	4.2 min	3.6 min
Depth of insertion	29.5 cm	21 cm
No discomfort	69%	29.6%
Mild–moderate discomfort	25.4%	50.7%
Severe discomfort	5.6%	19.7
Polyps detected	16	7

*Adapted from reference 3.

flexible examination, less than half were found with the rigid instrument.

COMPARISON OF 60-CM FLEXIBLE SIGMOIDOSCOPY WITH 35-CM FLEXIBLE SIGMOIDOSCOPY

We studied standard 60-cm flexible sigmoidoscopy versus 35-cm flexible sigmoidoscopy with respect to insertion distance, examination time, patient tolerance, and pathologic findings.[2] Since a potential important application of 35-cm flexible sigmoidoscopy might be the screening of patients for colorectal cancer and polyps, we studied 258 asymptomatic patients over the age of 45 with both instruments. Both sigmoidoscopes had 4-way tip deflection. Patients were examined sequentially by a single experienced examiner, with both 35-cm and 60-cm sigmoidoscopes. Patients were asked to rate their tolerance of each examination by a quantitative assessment of discomfort on a scale of 1 to 10 (1 = mildest; 10 = most severe) and to state which examination they preferred. The results are shown in Tables 7-2 and 7-3. Full insertion of the 35-cm instrument was achieved in nearly every patient in a mean time of 2.5 minutes, which was significantly shorter than the 60-cm examination time. Of 50 polypoid lesions found, 76% were seen with the 35-cm instrument, and 80% of patients with polyps had at least one visible with the shorter instrument. Patient tolerance of 35-cm sigmoidoscopy was better than 60-cm sigmoidoscopy, with only 29% having moderate or severe pain versus 69% with the longer instrument. Patient preference was 10 to 1 in favor of the shorter instrument.

Table 7-2
Insertion Distance, Examination Time, and Findings of 60-cm versus 35-cm Flexible Sigmoidoscopy*

	Sigmoidoscopy	
	35-cm	60-cm
Full insertion	98.5%	78.8%
Distance (mean)	34.9 cm	55.9%
Time (mean)	2.5 min	5.7 min
Total polyps seen	38/50 (76%)	49/50 (98%)
Total patients with polyps seen	31/39 (80%)	39/39 (100%)

*Adapted from reference 2.

Table 7-3
Patient Tolerance of 60-cm Versus 35-cm Flexible Sigmoidoscopy*

	Discomfort			
	Mild (1–3)	Moderate (4–7)	Severe (8–10)	Patient Preference
35-cm sigmoidoscopy	71%	21%	8%	72%
60-cm sigmoidoscopy	31%	49%	20%	7%

*Adapted from reference 2.

Zucker et al.[16] compared a slightly shorter 30-cm flexible sigmoido-scope to a 60-cm flexible sigmoidoscope in 96 consecutive symptomatic patients referred for sigmoidoscopy. The 30-cm examination was quicker (6.4 min versus 9.8 min), better tolerated, and found 82% (21 of 25) of the polypoid lesions that were seen with the 60-cm instrument. Inflam-matory bowel disease was seen nearly as often with the 30-cm instru-ment, but diverticulosis was documented more often with the 60-cm instrument.

These two studies clearly show that sigmoidoscopy with a shorter flexible instrument is a quicker and better tolerated examination that provides a very reasonable diagnostic yield of polypoid lesions and inflammatory bowel disease. Further evaluation is needed to determine whether the shorter instrument will be easier for the primary care phy-sician to incorporate safely and quickly into routine practice.

TRAINING PRIMARY CARE PHYSICIANS TO USE THE SHORTER FLEXIBLE SIGMOIDOSCOPE

Hocutt et al.[5] trained family physicians and family practice resi-dents to use the 35-cm flexible sigmoidoscope. The authors stated that *most* of the trainees learned to use the instrument effectively after 20 or less procedures.

Winawer et al.[15] trained a highly motivated primary care physician to use a 30-cm flexible sigmoidoscope. The learning process involved the following sequence (1) observation of flexible sigmoidoscopy and colonoscopy by an experienced endoscopist; (2) supervised experience with 30-cm flexible sigmoidoscopy in a colon model; (3) supervised patient examinations; (4) independent patient examinations; and (5) referral of patients with definite or questionable lesions to a supervising endoscopist for a repeat confirmatory examination with a 60-cm flexible sigmoidoscope. Within this carefully constructed teaching sequence, the trainee rapidly learned the insertion technique and achieved nearly full insertion of the instrument in 85% of cases. However, he required at least 50 examinations before he could reliably identify pathology, overcome problems with instrument insertion, and recognize suction artifacts. Examination time decreased from 8–12 or more minutes during the first 50 procedures to usually under 8 minutes during the next 150 examinations. Patient discomfort was minimal in over 75% of cases. Of the 22 polyps detected, 12 were between 17 and 30 cm from the anal verge and thus would be missed by standard rigid sigmoidoscopy.

It is apparent from this study that a motivated *nonendoscopist* can be adequately trained in the use of a 30-cm flexible sigmoidoscope. However, considerable time and effort was expended during both the training and quality control periods. It is possible that the motivated trainee might have achieved the same proficiency with a 60-cm flexible instrument during a similar training period. In addition, it is possible that once the physician mastered the technique necessary for 30-cm flexible sigmoidoscopy, he may have been able to use the longer 60-cm instrument. Weissman et al.[13] reported that during a multicenter study, several nonendoscopists quickly became proficient with a 30-cm flexible sigmoidoscope. After just 6–7 examinations under supervision the average depth of insertion was 27 cm with an average examination time of only 5.3 minutes and resulted in only minimal patient discomfort.

PROGRESSIVE TRAINING OF PRIMARY CARE PHYSICIANS IN USE OF THE 35-CM AND THEN THE 60-CM FLEXIBLE SIGMOIDOSCOPE

Schapiro et al.[11] reported their experience training community hospital primary care physicians and general surgeons in flexible sigmoidoscopy, initially with a 35-cm instrument followed by a 60-cm instrument. Seventy-five percent of physicians offered the program enrolled for training and 85% of these individuals completed an initial session, which included the use of a training model. However, only 10% of enrolled physicians completed the program. Reasons given for poor compliance by physicians in the program were (1) time commitment needed to become proficient; (2) rigid sigmoidoscopy was deemed adequate; (3) difficulty in submitting their private patients to a "training program;" and (4) concern about costs of the procedure and the instrument. However, some interesting findings were noted in physicians who completed the training program. These preceptors found that an an average of seven training sessions was sufficient to allow independent examination. Once proficient with a 35-cm instrument, only five additional supervised procedures were required for the trainee to become proficient with the 60-cm instrument. Finally, after completing the 35-cm instrument training session, some physicians purchased and independently became proficient with a 60-cm flexible sigmoidoscope.

Recently, American ACMI (Stamford, Connecticut) has marketed an overtube (see Chapter 5), which may allow for graded increases in distance of insertion during the training period. This 30-cm overtube or sleeve can be attached to a conventional 65-cm instrument, thus effectively limiting the examination to 35-cm. When both trainee and supervisor deem the time is right, the overtube can be easily removed and subsequent examinations performed to a full 60 cm.

The concept of progressive training with either a single instrument or with two of different lengths is an interesting one and needs further study. It is evident that major problems exist in adequately training nonendoscopists, including time constraints of both staff and trainees, solicitation of adequate numbers of patients, and convincing primary care physicians of the value of flexible sigmoidoscopy.

TRAINING PRIMARY CARE PHYSICIANS TO USE THE 60-CM FLEXIBLE SIGMOIDOSCOPE

Baskin et al.[1] trained 155 primary care physicians to use a 60-cm flexible sigmoidoscope. Four gastroenterologists supervised the trainee's procedures after each individual had completed 5 hours of didactic instruction, including review of videotape, slides, photographic atlases, and experience with endoscopic colon models. The trainees achieved a mean insertion distance of 49-cm, and mean examination time was 21 minutes. It was felt that a minimum experience of 25 cases with one-on-one supervision was necessary for the trainee to achieve competence.

Hawes and Lehman[4] trained 12 general medicine, surgery, and family practice residents to use a 60-cm flexible sigmoidoscope. They found that 25–30 procedures were required before most examinations were judged competent. They also noted that the trainees who had more experience with rigid sigmoidoscopy (more than 15 exams) attained competence earlier. Johnson et al.[6] in their Family Practice Training Program at UCLA, reported the training of 5 full-time faculty in the use of a 60-cm flexible sigmoidoscope by a gastroenterologist. The family practice staff in turn trained their residents in the use of the 60-cm sigmoidoscope. Between 1980 and 1982 more than 400 examinations were performed without complications.[7]

Rosevelt et al.[8] reported that a nurse practitioner, after an intensive training period, performed 825 flexible sigmoidoscopies independently with a 60-cm flexible sigmoidoscope. The nurse practitioner became quite proficient and reached an average insertion depth of 50 cm.

It is obvious that primary care physicians and paramedical persons can master either 35-cm or 60-cm flexible sigmoidoscopy. A massive expenditure of time and personnel would be required to train large numbers of such physicians in flexible sigmoidoscopy. More data is needed regarding the relative ease of learning flexible sigmoidoscopy, numbers of supervised examinations necessary, accuracy that can be achieved, and complications that may occur with the different instruments.

WHICH FLEXIBLE SIGMOIDOSCOPE SHOULD THE PRIMARY CARE PHYSICIAN USE?

Based on available data, which flexible sigmoidoscope should the primary care physician use? While the shorter 35-cm sigmoidoscope seems likely to be easier to master by nonendoscopist physicians and more tolerable for the patient, some polypoid lesions (~15–25%) will be missed. However, it appears that the 60-cm procedure can be taught to motivated physicians. Our current recommendations are that gastroenterologists, colorectal surgeons, and other physicians familiar with flexible endoscopy utilize 60-cm flexible sigmoidoscopy in their offices. Highly motivated nonendoscopists may learn and perform 60-cm flexible sigmoidoscopy, but the majority of primary care physicians should probably learn and implement 35-cm flexible sigmoidoscopy in their routine practice. The data suggests that a 35-cm instrument will detect at least twice as many polypoid lesions as the 25-cm rigid sigmoidoscope and should be considerably better tolerated by patients. Since the procedure duration is usually under 5 minutes, professional fees for 35-cm flexible sigmoidoscopy should approximate those for rigid sigmoidoscopy.

If a major shift in routine practice from rigid sigmoidoscopy to flexible sigmoidoscopy is to take place, a huge effort in training nonendoscopist physicians will be required. Training should optimally begin early, probably in the third or fourth year of medical school. The training of gastroenterology assistants and nurse practitioners is intriguing and may prove to be cost effective. Once a large cadre of flexible sigmoidoscopists exists, these individuals can train other physicians in their practice or hospital. For the immediate future, the leadership in teaching flexible sigmoidoscopy rests with the gastroenterologist and colorectal surgeon.

REFERENCES

1. Baskin WN, Greenlaw, RL, Frakes JT, et al.: Flexible sigmoidoscopy training for primary care physicians, Gastrointest Endosc (Abstract) 30:141, 1984.
2. Dubow RA, Katon RM, Benner KG, et al.: Short (35-cm.) vs. long (60-cm.) flexible sigmoidoscopy: A comparison of findings and tolerance in asymptomatic patients. Gastrointest Endosc (Abstract) 30:142, 1984.
3. Grobe JL, Kozarek RA, Sanowski RA: Flexible versus rigid sigmoidoscopy: A comparison using an inexpensive 35 cm flexible proctosigmoidoscope. Am J Gastroent 78:569–571, 1983.
4. Hawes R, Lehman G: Training resident physicians in fiberoptic sigmoidoscopy (FOS)—How many supervised examinations are needed? Gastrointest Endosc (Abstract) 30:143, 1984.
5. Hocutt JE, Jaffe R, Owens GM, Walters DT: 35-cm flexible fiberoptic sigmoidoscopy. Gastrointest Endosc (Abstract) 29:183, 1983.
6. Johnson RA, Quan M, Rodney WM: Flexible sigmoidoscopy in primary care. The procedure and its potential. Postgrad Med 72:151–154, 1982.
7. Johnson RA, Rodney WN, Quan M: Outcomes of flexible sigmoidoscopy in a family practice residency. J Fam Pract 15:785–789, 1982.
8. Rosevelt J, Frankl H: Colorectal cancer screening by nurse practitioner using a 60-cm flexible fiberoptic sigmoidoscope. Dig Dis Sci 29:161–163. 1984.
9. Sarles HE, Grobe JL, Sanowski RA: Use of a 35 cm flexible sigmoidoscope is practical and cost effective. Gastrointest Endosc (Abstract) 29:186, 1983.
10. Schapiro, M: Flexible sigmoidoscopy or short colonoscopy? Why settle for half of a loaf? Gastroenterology 77: 1156–1157, 1979.
11. Schapiro, M, Auslander MO, Getzug SJ, Klasky I: Flexible fiberoptic sigmoidoscopy training of non-endoscopic physicians in the community hospital. Gastrointest Endosc (Abstract) 29:186, 1983.
12. Tedesco FJ, Waye JD, Avella JR, Villalobos MM: Diagnostic implications of the spatial distribution of colonic mass lesions (polyps and cancers)— a prospective colonoscopic study. Gastrointest Endosc 26:95–97, 1980.
13. Weissman GS, Winawer SJ, Sergi H, et al.: Preliminary results of a multi-center evaluation of a 30 cm flexible sigmoidoscope. Gastrointest Endosc (Abstract) 28:150, 1982.
14. Who's for flexible sigmoidoscopy? Lancet (editorial) 2:893–894, 1983.
15. Winawer SJ, Cummins R, Baldwin MP, Ptak A: A new flexible sigmoidoscope for the generalist. Gastrointest Endosc 28:233–237, 1982.
16. Zucker GM, Madura MJ, Chmiel JS, Olinger EJ: The advantages of the 30-cm. flexible sigmoidoscope over the 60-cm flexible sigmoidoscope. Gastrointest Endosc 30:59–64, 1984.

8

Indications and Contraindications of Flexible Sigmoidoscopy Compared to Rigid Sigmoidoscopy and Colonoscopy

The indications for flexible sigmoidoscopy are controversial and continue to evolve. Several questions remain unresolved. When should flexible sigmoidoscopy be used in preference to standard rigid sigmoidoscopy? Should flexible fiberoptic sigmoidoscopes replace the rigid instruments? How does flexible sigmoidoscopy interface with colonoscopy? What will be the ultimate role of flexible sigmoidoscopy in general practice? This chapter will address these questions and review our interpretation of current indications for flexible sigmoidoscopy in comparison with rigid sigmoidoscopy and colonoscopy.

Despite clear evidence of superiority of flexible sigmoidoscopy over rigid sigmoidoscopy,[4,21] Haubrich stated in 1980, "My prediction is that the current wave of enthusiasm for flexible sigmoidoscopy will tend to ebb. I believe that flexible sigmoidoscopy eventually will be found to have a rather limited application."[10] In contrast with this prediction, interest in flexible sigmoidoscopy has grown steadily over the ensuing years, and numerous workshops are offered each year to teach this technique to general surgeons, family practitioners, and general internists. Indeed, in a 1982 symposium sponsored by the American Society for Gastrointestinal Endoscopy, Hogan[12] stated, "There is little doubt that flexible fiberoptic sigmoidoscopy will replace rigid sigmoidoscopy as the primary diagnostic instrument for detecting colorectal disease in the near future." Flexible sigmoidoscopy has, in fact, nearly replaced the rigid examination in the routine practice of most gastroenterologists and many colorectal surgeons. Use of flexible sigmoidoscopy by nonendoscopist practitioners, however, has been more limited, but a gradual transition from use of rigid to flexible instruments, particularly the 35-cm instrument, will likely occur in primary care practice over the next several years. A larger experience with 35-cm flexible sigmoidoscopy may necessitate future modification of the indications for sigmoidos-copy outlined in this chapter.

INDICATIONS FOR FLEXIBLE SIGMOIDOSCOPY

The indications for 35-cm and 60-cm flexible sigmoidoscopy are best reviewed in conjunction with the indications for rigid sigmoidos-copy and colonoscopy as shown in Table 8-1. The suspected anatomic area of colon involved with disease will generally dictate the procedure of choice. Table 8-1 is modified from the work of Hogan,[12] and will serve as the focus of this chapter. Each indication or group of indications for endoscopic visualization of the colon will be discussed in sequence, and the relative merits of each procedure will be reviewed.

Routine Use

Screening

The American Cancer Society recommends that individuals age 50 or older undergo a sigmoidoscopy yearly for 2 years, then every 3 to 5 years thereafter.[1] Rigid sigmoidoscopy may no longer be adequate to screen for polyps or carcinoma in an asymptomatic person. Several recent epidemiologic studies confirm a trend toward proximal migration of colorectal neoplasia.[28,29,33] Rigid sigmoidoscopy, at best, may discover only 25–35% of these lesions. The 35-cm flexible sigmoidoscope can increase this yield to perhaps 50–55%, and the 60-cm instrument to 65–70%. Colonoscopy, although much easier to perform with recent advances in instrumentation, remains too difficult, time consuming, and expen-sive to be considered a screening procedure. The ultimate screening procedure would be a "front-wheel drive" colonoscope, which would allow a 5-minute painless inspection of the colon! Colonoscopy will detect over 95% of all colonic lesions, but we are perhaps 10 years away from development of an instrument that will allow quick, safe, and painless inspection of the entire colon. For the present time, either the 35-cm or 60-cm flexible sigmoidoscopy appears to be the logical choice for screening asymptomatic patients.

Prior to Barium Enema

Most authorities continue to suggest that the rectum and sigmoid colon be inspected prior to barium enema examination.[12,20] However, it may now be reasonable to perform a barium enema first in a symptomatic patient to facilitate selection of the most appropriate endoscopic pro-cedure necessary to visualize the area in question in the colon. This latter approach may contain costs by avoiding flexible sigmoidoscopy in patients who will require subsequent colonoscopy based upon barium enema findings. On the other hand, sigmoidoscopy prior to barium enema can identify severe inflammatory bowel disease, which may contraindicate and defer barium studies, or detect the presence of a rectal or sigmoid obstructing lesion that would modify the technique of a barium enema. Although rigid sigmoidoscopy is adequate for rectal lesions, both 35-cm and 60-cm flexible sigmoidoscopy permit more proximal examination of the colon and are probably more desirable.

Rectal Bleeding

Stool Positive for Occult Blood

A positive test for occult blood in the stool indicates colonic neoplasia (polyps or cancer) in nearly 50% of patients.[38] Colonoscopy will provide the highest yield; however, if colonoscopy is not readily available, the combination of double-contrast barium enema and 60-cm flexible sigmoidoscopy will detect approximately 85% of polyps and 95–100% of cancers.[39] Rigid sigmoidoscopy plus standard barium enema will miss a significant number of lesions, particularly in the sigmoid colon, and is a much less acceptable work-up in this situation. Data are not yet available regarding the utility of 35-cm flexible sigmoidoscopy in this group of patients.

Stool Coated with Bright Red Blood

The history or finding of stool coated with a small amount of bright red blood nearly always signifies anorectal or left-sided colonic pathology. Careful anoscopy should be performed prior to or during sigmoidoscopy. If active disease (e.g., fissure, hemorrhoids, polyp, cancer, or proctitis) is located in the rectum, rigid sigmoidoscopy is adequate; however, the overall yield of pathology will be greater with 35-cm and 60-cm flexible sigmoidoscopy. Colonoscopy is only indicated when flexible sigmoidoscopy is negative.

Severe Rectal Bleeding

Several recent studies attest to the diagnostic efficacy of emergent colonoscopy for severe rectal bleeding after preliminary bowel preparation with an oral electrolyte preparation such as *Golytely*. The responsible lesion can be found in 70–85% of cases even in the presence of active bleeding.[5,14] In addition, a therapeutic maneuver may be employed during colonoscopy. For example, oozing arteriovenous malformations may be controlled by electrocoagulation or laser treatment, and bleeding polyps can be removed by snare cautery.[14] Some authors feel that patients with severe rectal bleeding should undergo initial panendoscopy, since

Table 8-1
Indications for Rigid Sigmoidoscopy, 35-cm Flexible Sigmoidoscopy, 60-cm Flexible Sigmoidoscopy, and Colonoscopy

| Indication | Sigmoidoscopy | | | Colonoscopy |
	Rigid	35-cm Flex	60-cm Flex	
Routine use				
Screening	2 + *	3 +	4 +	—
Prior to barium enema	2 +	3 +	4 +	—
Rectal bleeding				
Stool positive for occult blood	1 +	2 +	3 +	4 +
Stool coated with red blood	2 +	3 +	4 +	—
Severe hematochezia	1 +	2 +	2 +	4 +
Mass or stricture on barium enema				
Sigmoid or distal	—	2 +	4 +	—
Proximal to sigmoid	—	—	2 +	4 +
Colitis				
Inflammatory bowel disease	2 +	3 +	4 +	—
Infectious colitis	4 +	4 +	4 +	—
Ischemic colitis	—	2 +	4 +	—

Radiation-induced colitis	2+	3+	—
Antibiotic-associated colitis	2+	3+	—
Proctitis	4+	2+	—
Ileostomy dysfunction	—	4+	—
Diverticular disease			
Left-sided	—	2+	—
Right-sided	—	—	4+
Surveillance			
In ulcerative colitis	—	—	4+
After resection of polyps and cancer	—	—	4+
Miscellaneous conditions			
Acquired immune deficiency syndrome (AIDS)	4+	2+	2+
Solitary rectal ulcer	4+	2+	—
Submucosal biopsies	4+	—	—
Acute distal colonic obstruction	1+	2+	—
Sigmoid volvulus decompression	4+	?	3+ (?)
Decompression of acute nontoxic megacolon	—	—	4+

Modified from Hogan.[5]

*The rating scale summarizes the relative strength of the indication for each endoscopic procedure as follows: — = not indicated; 1+ = least indicated; 2–3+ = moderately indicated; 4+ = most indicated.

10–15% of these patients are bleeding from an upper gastrointestinal source such as peptic ulcer. Occasionally, severe hemorrhage originates from the rectum or sigmoid colon and can be diagnosed by rigid or flexible sigmoidoscopy.

Mass or Stricture on Barium Enema

The anatomic level of a lesion seen on a barium enema will dictate the endoscopic procedure necessary to evaluate the abnormal area. Disease of the sigmoid colon is usually well seen with the 60-cm flexible sigmoidoscope. In our flexible sigmoidoscopy study[15] of patients with sigmoid colon abnormalities, 14 had a suspected sigmoid stricture and 11 of these had a specific diagnosis made by flexible sigmoidoscopy, while no stricture was found in 3 patients. The rigid and 35-cm flexible sigmoidoscopes will not reliably reach radiographically-detected lesions in the sigmoid colon. Abnormalities well above the sigmoid colon (mid-descending or proximal colon) are better evaluated by colonoscopy, since the 60-cm instrument cannot reliably reach those levels.

Colitis

Inflammatory Bowel Disease

While ulcerative colitis involves the rectum in nearly 100% of cases, Crohn's disease of the colon spares the rectum approximately 50% of the time. Therefore, sigmoidoscopes of increased length will detect a greater proportion of Crohn's disease patients. Endoscopists should be cautious when performing sigmoidoscopy in patients with severe colitis and avoid bowel preparations, which could precipitate toxic megacolon. Air insufflation should be kept to a minimum, and there is usually no need to examine the bowel higher than the rectum when it is abnormal. If the rectum is involved, the degree of inflammation will usually be representative of the rest of the colon and the full extent of the disease can be determined at a later date.

If inflammatory bowel disease is still suspected after a normal flexible sigmoidoscopy to 60 cm, then colonoscopy is indicated. Crohn's disease may be segmental and often is limited to the proximal colon. In addition, expert colonoscopists can often (25–50%) intubate the ileum and determine if there is terminal ileal disease.

Infectious Colitis

Infectious colitis accounts for approximately 40% of newly diagnosed cases of acute bloody diarrhea.[36] Campylobacter is generally the most commonly isolated pathogen in the United States, followed by

Shigella, Salmonella, and *Entamoeba histolytica.* Some organisms, such as *Shigella,* nearly always involve the rectum, while others, such as *E. histolytica,* may or may not affect the rectum. Amebiasis most frequently involves the cecum and ascending colon and less frequently the descending and sigmoid colon or rectum. When rectal involvement is present in infectious colitis, the abnormalities seen during sigmoidoscopy are nonspecific and usually atypical for inflammatory bowel disease. Mucosal findings include patchy petechial hemorrhages and focal areas of erythematous, edematous, and granular mucosa.[36] Diagnosis can be made equally as well with rigid, 35-cm or 60-cm flexible sigmoidoscopy. Colonoscopy is generally not indicated and may be harmful if inflammation is severe.

Ischemic Colitis

Scowcroft et al.[32] described the usual anatomic distribution of ischemic colitis observed during colonoscopy. Twelve of 15 patients (80%) would be diagnosed by 60-cm flexible sigmoidoscopy, but only 5 of 15 patients (33%) with standard rigid sigmoidoscopy. Since diagnosis is usually established with flexible sigmoidoscopy, full colonoscopy is not generally indicated. In acute ischemic colitis, there is edema, spasm, and often severe friability similar to ulcerative colitis (see Chapter 11, Fig. 11-4). In the resolving stage, deep ulcers, similar to those seen in Crohn's disease, may be seen. Flexible sigmoidoscopy should be performed gently or avoided if peritoneal signs, high fever, and leukocytosis are present.

Radiation-Induced Colitis

Radiation-induced colitis is a relatively frequent sequellae of pelvic irradiation therapy for carcinoma of the cervix, bladder, ovary, vagina, or prostate. It may develop as early as 3 months or as late as 20 years following treatment.[27] The usual manifestations are rectal bleeding and/or partial sigmoid obstruction. Barium enema often shows a sigmoid stricture. Although the rectum is often involved, marked fixation and angulation of the sigmoid colon usually makes rigid sigmoidoscopy difficult and even hazardous.[27] Flexible sigmoidoscopy is preferable, with the 60-cm instrument probably providing greater yield than the 35-cm sigmoidoscope. Gross mucosal changes include edema, friability, superficial ulceration, and a very characteristic pattern of large telangiectatic vessels (see Chapter 11, Fig. 11-12).

Antibiotic-Associated (Pseudomembranous) Colitis

This entity produces a characteristic endoscopic picture of whitish-yellow plaques on an edematous mucosa (see Chapter 11, Fig. 10). The plaques are very adherent and result in petechial bleeding points when wiped off. Tedesco et al.[35] showed that rectal sparing occurs in 23% of cases but that only 9% are missed by 60-cm flexible sigmoidoscopy. Thus the 60-cm flexible sigmoidoscope is probably the instrument of choice when antibiotic-associated colitis is suspected.

Proctitis

Proctitis may be idiopathic (see Chapter 11, Fig. 11-6) and nonspecific or caused by a number of venereal agents such as *Neisseria gonorrhea, Treponema pallidum, Chlamydia,* and others.[34] After a specific diagnosis is made with appropriate biopsies, swabs, and cultures, treatment may be instituted. Swabbing inflamed or ulcerated mucosa or collecting liquid stool for culture and sensitivity are best performed through the rigid sigmoidoscope. Follow-up can also be performed easily with rigid sigmoidoscopy.

Ileostomy Dysfunction or Disease

Patients with ileostomies or colostomies for ulcerative colitis, Crohn's disease, or carcinoma may develop new gastrointestinal symptoms. Inspection of the ileum or colon can be accomplished easily through the stoma of the ostomy by endoscopy with the flexible sigmoidoscope, and biopsies of suspected inflammation or neoplasm can be obtained. Rigid instruments are unsatisfactory for these examinations because of the usual sharp postoperative bowel angulations, and examination by colonoscopy is usually unnecessary.

The continent ileostomy[17] (Kock pouch) is becoming more widely employed as an alternative to the standard Brooke ileostomy after total colectomy for ulcerative colitis. About 10% of these patients develop ileostomy dysfunction. Waye et al.[37] were successful in studying the bowel of these patients with flexible sigmoidoscopes and even performed electrosurgery for an adhesive band in one and removed a foreign body in another. These patients may also develop an entity called *pouch ileitis*,[16] which presents with bloody diarrhea, fever, and weight loss. Bacterial overgrowth in the pouch is the probable etiology of this syndrome, and therapy with metronidazole often leads to resolution. Diagnosis and follow-up is best performed with a flexible sigmoidoscope.

Diverticular Disease

Left-sided diverticular disease (see Chapter 11, Fig. 11-13) is most often symptomatic either from a microperforation of a diverticulum and diverticulitis, or from muscular hypertrophy with obstructive symptoms.[13,23] The clinical picture and/or barium enema is often inconclusive, and the differentiation from carcinoma, ischemic colitis, and Crohn's disease can be difficult. Furthermore, polypoid lesions or cancer are easily missed radiographically in an area of extensive sigmoid colon diverticulosis. The rigid sigmoidoscope rarely reaches the area of involvement,[10] and the 35-cm flexible sigmoidoscope fails to reach left-sided diverticula in about one-third of cases.[7] The 60-cm flexible instrument is preferred for more complete sigmoid colon visualization.[7,39] Sigmoidoscopy should be performed with extreme care, minimal air insufflation, and very gentle advancement when diverticulitis is suspected. If peritoneal signs are present, it is best to defer sigmoidoscopy and treat with antibiotics until clinical improvement is evident.

Right-sided diverticular disease is only rarely associated with acute diverticulitis. However, most diverticular hemorrhage (60–70%) arises from right-sided diverticula.[8] When active bleeding or other suspected complications from right-sided diverticula occur, full colonoscopy is obviously indicated.

Surveillance
Ulcerative colitis

It is well recognized that long-standing ulcerative colitis is associated with a high incidence of colonic cancer.[19] Risk factors for cancer include extent of disease (universal colitis has the greatest risk), duration of disease (8–10 years or longer), and perhaps continuous activity. The finding of severe dysplasia by colonic biopsy of abnormal mucosa or a slightly elevated plaque-like lesion is an indication for consideration of total colectomy, because 30–50% of these patients have colonic cancer, which is often not grossly detectable by colonoscopy or barium enema.[6,3] Colonoscopic surveillance with multiple biopsies should begin 8–10 years after the onset of universal colitis and 15–20 years after the presence of left-sided colitis. Dysplasia may be patchy in distribution and spares the left colon in at least 25–30% of cases. Therefore, rigid and flexible sigmoidoscopy are inadequate for surveillance, and total colonoscopy is mandatory. The optimal frequency of colonoscopy has not been established but probably should be performed annually or every other year.

After Resection of Polyps or Cancer

Metachronous lesions occur frequently following polypectomy or resection of colon cancer.[40] Polyps recur in 20–30% of cases, and new colon cancers develop in 3–5% of individuals. In addition, the colonic anastomosis after cancer resection may be the site of tumor recurrence. Rigid or flexible sigmoidoscopy are not acceptable follow-up procedures for these patients, because recurrent polyps or cancer may occur anywhere in the colon. Full colonoscopy should be performed at initial diagnosis and repeated in one year. Thereafter, occult fecal blood tests should be performed yearly and either colonoscopy or flexible sigmoidoscopy, plus double-contrast barium enema, performed every three years.

Miscellaneous

Acquired Immune Deficiency Syndrome (AIDS)

Diarrhea is a frequent occurrence in patients with AIDS and is often related to viral or bacterial proctitis or colitis. Their colon may also be the site of Kaposi's sarcoma. Patients with suspected or confirmed AIDS who are referred for proctosigmoidoscopy should preferably have rigid sigmoidoscopy with a disposable instrument until more is known about the agent(s) responsible for this disease. If a flexible sigmoidoscopy or colonoscopy is required on a patient who has AIDS, the instrument should be gas sterilized. Some units have available a "dedicated" fiberoptic instrument which is used only on AIDS patients. The examiner should also take special precautions during examination and use gloves, gown, and masks.

Solitary Rectal Ulcer

This condition is characterized by a large, deep, indolent rectal ulcer of unknown etiology.[30] Initial biopsies should be taken to rule out specific diseases such as carcinoma, lymphoma, Crohn's disease, tuberculosis, or amebiasis. Once the diagnosis is established, follow-up of the ulcer can be achieved conveniently with rigid sigmoidoscopy.

Submucosal Biopsies

Certain diseases with predominant submucosal involvement, such as amyloidosis,[18] Crohn's disease,[11] lymphoma,[26] and Hirschsprung's,[22] may be established by deep, submucosal rectal biopsy. Biopsy forceps used during flexible sigmoidoscopy limit the depth of the tissue specimen to the mucosa only and are much less useful in establishing the diagnosis in these conditions. Biopsies obtained with the rigid forceps should be taken below the peritoneal reflection (<10-cm from anal verge) and from the face of a lower rectal valve if possible to reduce the chance of perforation. Both bleeding and perforation can occur, and this technique should be performed by experienced examiners.

Acute Distal Large Bowel Obstruction

A suspected distal large bowel obstruction may be documented by performing a cautious barium enema, with care taken not to fill the proximal colon with barium. A gentle flexible sigmoidoscopy, preferably with the 60-cm instrument, may also be attempted and may be helpful to obtain biopsies if a mass lesion or stricture is noted.

Sigmoid Volvulus Decompression

Gentle decompression of a sigmoid volvulus is successful in 51–77% of cases using a rigid sigmoidoscope.[9,2] There are recent reports of success with a colonoscope[31] and with a 60-cm flexible sigmoidoscope.[25]

Decompression of Acute Nontoxic Megacolon (Ogilvie's Syndrome)

There are many causes of an acute nontoxic megacolon in adults. This syndrome occurs most often in acutely ill elderly patients after surgery or trauma. The colon rapidly dilates and, when the cecum reaches approximately 12-cm in diameter, perforation may occur. Surgical decompression is hazardous in these elderly and ill patients. Decompression has been performed by colonoscopy, but it is an extremely difficult procedure and should be employed by only the expert colonoscopist.[24] Shorter instruments are probably ineffective.

CONTRAINDICATIONS TO FLEXIBLE SIGMOIDOSCOPY

There are only a few contraindications to flexible sigmoidoscopy and they are relative, depending upon the importance of the potential information to be acquired. Standard contraindications to flexible sigmoidoscopy are acute peritonitis, fulminant colitis (any etiology), acute, severe diverticulitis, toxic megacolon, large aortic aneurysm, and an uncooperative patient.

Indications and containdications for both 60-cm and 35-cm flexible sigmoidoscopy will be in a state of flux for several years as these instruments become more widely employed by a greater variety of physicians. It is important for the primary care physician to know the indications for colonoscopy in order to facilitate diagnosis and limit duplication of tests or failure to make a diagnosis. Indications for rigid sigmoidoscopy are relatively limited to conditions where only the rectum needs to be visualized, deep mucosal biopsies or swabs for cultures are desired, or AIDS is suspected. The information provided in this chapter is meant to be a comparative guideline for the application of the endoscopic procedures that are currently available to assess colorectal disorders.

REFERENCES

1. American Cancer Society: Cancer of the colon and rectum. CA 30:208–215, 1980.

2. Arnold GJ, Nance FC: Volvulus of the sigmoid colon. Ann Surg 177:527–537, 1973.
3. Blackstone MO, Riddell RH, Rogers BHG, Levin B: Dysplasia-associated lesion or mass (DALM) detected by colonoscopy in long-standing ulcerative colitis. An indication for colectomy. Gastroenterology 80:366–374, 1981.
4. Bohlman TW, Katon RM, Lipshutz GR, et al.: Fiberoptic pansigmoidoscopy. An evaluation and comparison with rigid sigmoidoscopy. Gastroenterology 72:644–649, 1977.
5. Caos A, Manier J, Benner K, et al.: "Golytely" preparation for colonoscopy in acute lower gastrointestinal hemorrhage. Gastrointest Endosc (Abstract) 29:157, 1983.
6. Dobbins WO: Current status of the precancer lesion in ulcerative colitis. Gastroenterology 73:1431–1433, 1977.
7. Dubow RA, Katon RM, Benner KG, et al.: Short (35-cm) vs. long (60-cm) flexible sigmoidoscopy: A comparison of findings and tolerance in asymptomatic patients. Gastrointest Endosc (Abstract) 30:142, 1984.
8. Eisenberg H. Laufer I, Skillman JJ: Arteriographic diagnosis and management of suspected colonic diverticular hemorrhage. Gastroenterology 64:1091–1100, 1973.
9. Greenlee HB, Pienbos EJ, Vanderbilt PC, et al.: Acute large bowel obstruction. Arch Surg 108:470–476, 1974.
10. Haubrich WS: Comments relevant to rigid proctosigmoidoscopy, flexible fiberoptic sigmoidoscopy, and colonoscopy. Gastrointest Endosc 26:18s–19s, 1980.
11. Hill RB, Kent TH, Hansen RN: Clinical usefulness of rectal biopsy in Crohn's disease. Gastroenterology 77:938–944, 1979.
12. Hogan WJ: Flexible sigmoidoscopy versus colonoscopy—when to use which instrument. Gastrointest Endosc 29:126–128, 1982.
13. Hughes LE: Complications of diverticular disease: inflammation, obstruction and bleeding. Clin Gastroenterol 4:147–170, 1975.
14. Jensen DM, Machicado GA, Tapia JI: Emergent colonoscopy in patients with severe hematochezia. Gastrointest Endosc (Abstract) 29:177, 1983.
15. Katon RM, Melnyk CS: The pansigmoidoscope: One year's experience in a gastrointestinal dianostic unit. J Clin Gastroent 1:41–45, 1979.
16. Klein K, Stenzel P, Katon RM: Pouch ileitis: Report of a case with severe systemic manifestations. J Clin Gastroent 5:149–154, 1983.
17. Kock NG: Ileostomy without external appliance. Ann Surg 173:545–550, 1971.
18. Kyle RA, Bayrd ED: Amyloidosis: Review of 236 cases. Medicine 54:271–299, 1975.
19. Lennard-Jones JE, Morson BC, Ritchie JC, et al.: Cancer in colitis: Assessment of the individual risk by clinical and histological criteria. Gastroenterology 73:1280–1289, 1977.
20. Manier J: The role of flexible sigmoidoscopy in the practice of a gastroenterologist. 29:122–123, 1983.
21. Marks G, Boggs W, Castro AF, et al.: Sigmoidoscopic examination with rigid and flexible fiberoptic sigmoidoscopes in the surgeon's office. A compara-

tive perspective study of effectiveness in 1,012 cases. Dis Colon Rectum 22:162–168, 1979.

22. Morikawa Y, Donahue PK, Hendren WH: Manometry and histochemistry in the diagnosis of Hirschsprung's disease. Pediatrics 63:865–871, 1979.

23. Morson BC: Pathology of diverticular disease of the colon. Clin Gastroenterol 4:37–52, 1975.

24. Norton L, Young D, Scribner R: Management of pseudo-obstruction of the colon. Surg Gynecol Obstet 138:595–598, 1974.

25. O'Connor JJ: Reduction of sigmoid volvulus by flexible sigmoidoscope. Arch Surg 114:1092, 1979.

26. Quan SHQ: Uncommon malignant anal and rectal tumors, in Stearns MW, Jr. (Ed.), Neoplasms of the Colon, Rectum and Anus. New York: John Wiley & Sons, 1980, pp 115–142.

27. Reichelderfer M, Morrissey JF: Colonoscopy in radiation colitis. Gastrointest Endosc 26:41–43, 1980.

28. Rhodes JB, Holmes FF, Clark GM: Changing distribution patterns of primary cancers in the large bowel. JAMA 238:641–643, 1977.

29. Rosato FE, Marks G: Changing site distribution patterns of colorectal cancer at Thomas Jefferson University Hospital. Dis Colon Rectum 24:93–95, 1981.

30. Rutter KRP, Riddel RH: The solitary ulcer syndrome of the rectum. Clin Gastroenterol 4:505–530, 1975.

31. Sanner CJ, Saltzman DA: Detorsion of sigmoid volvulus by colonoscopy. Gastrointest Endosc 23:212–213, 1977.

32. Scowcroft CW, Sanowski RA, Kozarek RA: Colonoscopy in ischemic colitis. Gastrointest Endosc 27:156–161, 1981.

33. Snyder DN, Hester JF, Meigs JW, Flannery JT: Changes in site distribution of colorectal carcinoma in Connecticut, 1940–1973. Dig Dis Sci 22:791–797, 1977.

34. Sohn N, Robelitti JG: The gay bowel syndrome, a review of colonic and rectal conditions in 200 male homosexuals. Am J Gastroenterology 67:478–484, 1977.

35. Tedesco FJ, Corless JK, Brownstein RE: Rectal sparing in antibiotic associated pseudomembranous colitis: A prospective study. Gastroenterology 83:1259–1260, 1982.

36. Tedesco JF, Hardin RD, Harper RN, Edwards BH: Infectious colitis endoscopically simulating inflammatory bowel disease: A prospective evaluation. Gastrointest Endosc 29:195–197, 1983.

37. Waye JD, Kreel I, Bauer J, Gelernt IM: The continent ileostomy: Diagnosis and treatment of problems by means of operative fiberoptic endoscopy. Gastrointest Endosc 23:196–198, 1977.

38. Winawer SJ, Fleisher M, Baldwin M, Sherlock P: Current status of fecal occult blood testing in screening for colorectal cancer. CA 32:100–112, 1982.

39. Winawer SJ, Leidner SD, Boyle C, Kurtz RC: Comparison of flexible sigmoidoscopy with other diagnostic techniques in the diagnosis of rectocolon neoplasia. Dig Dis Sci 24:277–281, 1979.

40. Winawer SJ, Sherlock P, Schottenfeld D, Miller DG: Screening for colon cancer. Gastroenterology 70:783–789, 1976.

9

Potential Complications of Flexible
Sigmoidoscopy and Polypectomy

Flexible sigmoidoscopy is a relatively recent addition to the armamentarium of the endoscopist. Since our study of flexible sigmoidoscopy in 1977,[4] numerous series comprising over 10,000 cases have been reported.[10,17-20,23,25,29-31,33,44,45,47,49,50] Only one major complication of flexible sigmoidoscopy, a case of colonic perforation, has been reported to date.[30] This incidence of perforation (0.01%) seems very low when compared to diagnostic colonoscopy, which has a reported average perforation rate of 1 in 500 cases (0.2%) (Table 9-1).[2,15,16,28,40,43]

There is no room for complacency, however, since most series of flexible sigmoidoscopy have been reported by endoscopists experienced in the technique and hazards of colonoscopy. The new generation of flexible sigmoidoscopists in general medical and surgical practices will not likely be as attuned to the hazards of negotiating the sigmoid colon, particularly in patients with diverticular disease, strictures, and postoperative adhesions. In addition, although only one reported perforation exists in the literature, we are aware of additional unreported cases over the last two years. Therefore, the literature does not represent the true incidence of the complications of flexible sigmoidoscopy.

The potential for all complications of diagnostic colonoscopy exists with flexible sigmoidoscopy. The risk will likely be lower than with colonoscopy, but only data from large surveys of flexible sigmoidoscopy will determine the true risk of this procedure. The data published in the literature regarding the complications of colonoscopy will be reviewed in this chapter. Full understanding of the complications of colonoscopy is essential to minimize accidents during flexible sigmoidoscopy.

Incidence of Perforation by Diagnostic Colonoscopy

Author*	Cases (No.)	Perforations (No.)	Deaths (No.)
Rogers[40]	25,298	55	2
Gilbert[16]	700	1	1
Macrae[28]	5,000	4	0
Berci[2]	3,850	7	0
Geenan[15]	814	7	0
Smith[43]	6,290	5	1
Totals	41,952	79 (0.19%)	4

*First author and reference number.

COMPLICATIONS OF DIAGNOSTIC COLONOSCOPY

Perforation

The reported incidence of perforation complicating diagnostic colonoscopy is low and averages about one per 500 cases (Table 9-1). Clinical conditions that predispose patients to an increased risk for colonic perforation (Table 9-2) should be recognized and a more cautious approach taken during the procedure. During flexible endoscopy of the colon, perforation is most likely to occur in the sigmoid colon, where sharp angulations may develop in a redundant bowel. In one large study where the site of perforation was stated, the sigmoid colon was involved in nearly 80% of the cases.[40]

Mechanisms of Perforation

Perforation may occur from either mechanical or pneumatic pressure.

Mechanical perforation A particular risk of mechanical perforation exists in the conditions listed in Table 9-2. In diverticulosis, the bowel wall is hypertrophic and poorly distensible, resulting in a narrowed lumen. When multiple and large diverticular orifices are present, the endoscopist may mistake a diverticular orifice for the bowel lumen and cause rupture of the thin diverticular sac by either pneumatic pressure or mechanical pressure from the advancing instrument tip (Fig. 9-1). Acute diverticulitis has the additional factors of edema, further

Conditions that Predispose Patients to an Increased
Risk of Perforation at Colonoscopy

- Diverticulosis and diverticulitis

- Previous pelvic surgery with adhesions

- Pelvic inflammatory disease

- Previous pelvic irradiation therapy

- Severe inflammatory bowel disease

- Ischemic bowel disease

- Sigmoid colon strictures

luminal narrowing, and often a mass effect. Since acute diverticulitis usually represents a walled-off colonic microperforation, flexible sigmoidoscopy is contraindicated until clinical improvement is evident.

Previous pelvic surgery or pelvic inflammatory disease may cause extensive adhesions, and make the sigmoid colon stiff, unyielding and more acutely angulated. In this situation, the sigmoid colon is often not negotiable despite maximal tip deflection, torque, and other insertion maneuvers. Excessive force by the shaft of the flexible instrument may cause a mechanical perforation (Fig. 9-2).

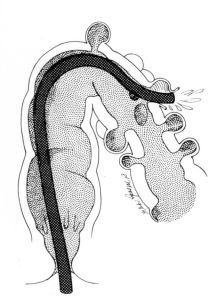

Mechanical perforation. Sigmoidoscope tip inadvertantly entering a large diverticular orifice and perforating a diverticulum.

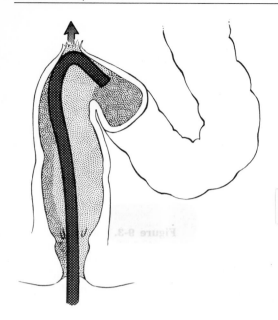

Mechanical perforation. Sharply angulated sigmoidoscope shaft becoming the leading edge, and excessive force causes the shaft to perforate the sigmoid colon (*dark arrow*).

The irradiated colon and active inflammatory bowel disease may be associated with thinning and weakness of the bowel wall. In these cases, even the usual amount of mechnical pressure may occasionally result in perforation.

Finally, strictures of the bowel may be caused by necrotic tumor, ulcerating lesions (e.g., Crohn's disease), or surgical anastomoses. Overzealous attempts to force the instrument tip through such narrowed areas may lead to direct mechnical perforation. (Fig. 9-3)

Pneumatic perforation   Although most colonic perforations at colonoscopy are the result of direct mechanical pressure from the instrument shaft and tip, insufflated air can lead to overdistention of the colonic wall and perforation. Even though the flexible sigmoidoscope does not reach beyond the sigmoid or descending colon, pneumatic pressure may lead to perforation in the transverse colon, ascending colon, or cecum.

Fortunately, pneumatic perforation is uncommon, since excess gas is usually refluxed into the terminal ileum or passed rectally (Fig. 9-4A). Burt[7] found the rectum to be the most resistant to pneumatic rupture, followed by the sigmoid colon, transverse colon, and cecum. The cecum is most susceptible to pneumatic perforation since it has the thinnest wall and greatest diameter. Studies by Kozarek et al.[21] in human cadavers found that the cecum ruptured at a mean intraluminal pressure

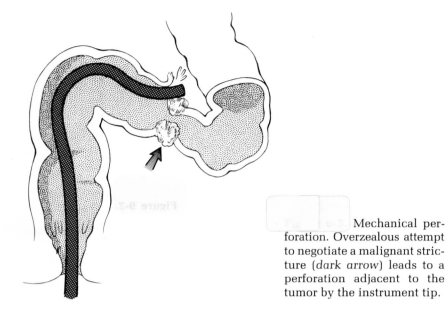

Mechanical perforation. Overzealous attempt to negotiate a malignant stricture (*dark arrow*) leads to a perforation adjacent to the tumor by the instrument tip.

of 81 mmHg, while the sigmoid required a much higher pressure of 169 mmHg, for rupture. Insufflated air usually escapes via the ileocecal valve and/or rectum (Fig. 9-4A), but a cecal perforation or serosal laceration can occur in a patient with a competent ileocecal valve or ileal disease when the tip of the scope is impacted in a stricture (Fig. 9-4B). High intraluminal pressures may also result when air is insufflated while the instrument tip is impacted against the wall of the bowel, as in the slide-by maneuver.[21] To avoid pneumatic perforation during flexible sigmoidoscopy, air insufflation should be used sparingly, particularly when the instrument tip is impacted against the wall or is in a stricture.

Anatomic Types of Perforation

Perforation may occur freely into the peritoneal cavity, may be closed into the retroperitoneum, or may be occult and benign (Table 9-3). Each of these varieties of perforation, and also transmural injury in the form of serosal lacerations, are discussed.

Free perforation   This form of perforation is the most common and complicates from 1/200 to 1/1,000 diagnostic colonoscopies.[27] It is immediately obvious to the endoscopist by direct visualization of the peritoneal cavity in many cases.[2,15,16,28,40,43] On occasion a delayed perforation[12] occurs several days after the procedure. Physical examination reveals abdominal distention, a quiet abdomen, and loss of hepatic

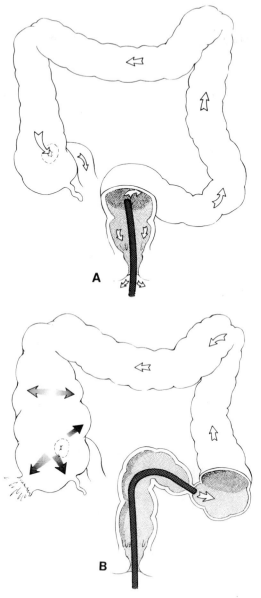

Figure 8-3. Pneumatic perforation. (A) Normally, insufflated air can escape rectally and via ileocecal valve (*arrows*). (B) Sigmoidoscope tip impacted in stricture—no escape of air via rectum or into the ileum through a competent ileocecal valve, resulting in cecal perforation (dark arrows).

Table 9-3
Types of Perforation and Bowel Injury at Colonoscopy or Polypectomy

	Diagnosis	Treatment	Prognosis
Free perforation	• Severe abdominal pain; distention • Signs of peritoneal irritation, loss of hepatic dullness, fever, leukocytosis • Abdominal film: free intraperitoneal air • Endoscopic visualization of peritoneum	NPO* IV fluids Antibiotics *Urgent laparotomy*—primary closure of rent in colon	5 percent mortality
Retroperitoneal perforation	• Abdominal pain, distention • Subcutaneous emphysema (scrotum, chest, neck) • Low-grade fever, leukocytosis • Abdominal film: subcutaneous air • Chest x-ray: mediastinal air	NPO IV fluids Antibiotics Close clinical observation Laparotomy not usually indicated	Gradual improvement over 7–8 days Rare mortality
Benign pneumoperitoneum	• Asymptomatic or mild distention • Low-grade fever • Abdominal film: free intraperitoneal air	NPO IV fluids Antibiotics	Rapid improvement over 2–3 days No mortality
Serosal lacerations	• Asymptomatic or abdominal pain and/or distention • Afebrile • Abdominal film: normal	NPO IV fluids	Rapid improvement over 2–3 days No mortality
Post-polypectomy coagulation syndrome	• Localized abdominal pain • Peritoneal irritation, fever, leukocytosis • Abdominal film: normal	NPO IV fluids Antibiotics Rarely requires laparotomy	Rapid improvement over 2–4 days Rare mortality

*NPO = nothing by mouth.

110

dullness. A plain abdominal film shows massive intraperitoneal air. Fever and leukocytosis are common. Most patients are managed successfully with intravenous fluids, antibiotics, and urgent exploratory laporatomy to repair the rent in the colon, usually by debridement and primary closure.[40] The prognosis is relatively good, with a reported mortality rate of 5%. The prior colonoscopic preparation reduces bacterial and fecal contamination of the peritoneum and makes for a relatively sterile environment. Bowel preparation is not nearly as complete with flexible sigmoidoscopy (1 or 2 Phospho-Soda enemas), and thus a greater potential for peritoneal contamination and resultant complications exists.

Retroperitoneal (closed) perforation   This type of perforation is relatively rare and is probably more common with pneumatic than with mechanical perforation. It may not be obvious at the time of endoscopy but may present after colonoscopy with subcutaneous air enlarging the scrotum or passing through the mediastinum into the neck. Abdominal and chest x-rays will disclose retroperitoneal and subcutaneous air.[24] Patients with closed perforation usually have abdominal pain, distention, low-grade fever, and leukocytosis. Most patients can be managed conservatively with intravenous fluids and antibiotics, and clinical and radiographic improvement occurs over several days. Surgery is usually not necessary. This type of perforation has been seen with both diagnostic colonoscopy[24] and colonoscopic polypectomy.[51]

Benign pneumoperitoneum   Echer et al.[13] studied 100 consecutive patients undergoing both diagnostic and therapeutic colonoscopy. Routine post-procedure abdominal films disclosed one patient with extensive free intraperitoneal air. The patient remained asymptomatic but developed a fever of 38.1°C and was treated conservatively with intravenous fluid and antibiotics. The free air decreased slowly over the next 72 hours. Others have noted the same phenomenon, which is thought to represent tiny leaks through the bowel wall.

Serosal laceration (incomplete perforation)   Serosal tears in the colon have been described both following standard colonoscopy[26] and intraoperative colonoscopy.[42] Serosal or seromuscular tears are most common in the sigmoid colon, where they are thought to result from mechanical pressure. Cecal lacerations can also occur, probably due to pneumatic pressure. In the experimental animal, increasing intraluminal pressure results in sequential seromuscular stripping, mucosal laceration, and finally mucosal rupture. This progressive injury occurs along the longitudinal bands of the antimesenteric wall of the colon (Fig. 9-5). Factors contributing to serosal and seromuscular tears during colonoscopy are (1) a large volume of air; (2) rapid insufflation of air;

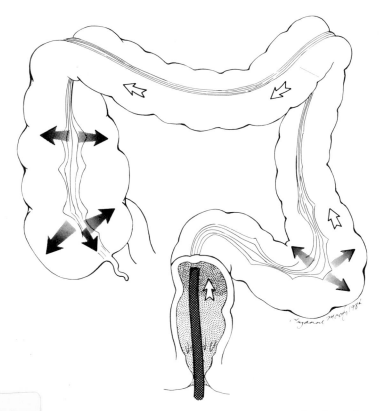

Figure 9-5. Serosal laceration—Tears occur most commonly along the antimesenteric wall of the sigmoid colon or cecum (*dark arrows*).

(3) compartmentalization of the insufflated air; and (4) localized mechanical stretching and bowing of the antimesenteric wall of the sigmoid colon during instrument insertion.

Clinically, the patient may be asymptomatic (tears have been observed at operative colonoscopy) or develop abdominal pain and distention following colonoscopy. Management consists of intravenous fluids and withholding oral feedings for 48–72 hours.

Hemorrhage

This complication is much less common than perforation, occurring in less than 1/1000 cases.[27] Hemorrhage is usually minor and may develop by mechanical irritation of an inflamed colon or occur after colonic biopsy. Caution should be exerted when performing flexible sigmoidos-copy in patients with severe inflammatory bowel disease. If a coagulo-pathy is suspected, a platelet count, bleeding time, and prothrombin time should be available prior to biopsy. Major hemorrhage is much more common after colonic polypectomy, which will be discussed later in this chapter.

Cardiopulmonary Complications

Major cardiopulmonary events are very rare and occur in 1 of 2500 cases.[27]

Pulmonary

The pulmonary complications of colonoscopy are limited to those associated with medications. The American Society for Gastrointestinal Endoscopy survey of over 25,000 cases of diagnostic colonoscopy reported 8 patients with respiratory depression secondary to medication, includ-ing 5 respiratory arrests.[40] Since flexible sigmoidoscopy does not usually require sedation, respiratory complications should be extremely rare.

Cardiac

Hypotension   A fall in blood pressure may occur from medication or as the result of a vasovagal response secondary to colonic distention with air and/or mechanical pressure. Usually, vasovagal hypotension is not serious and responds rapidly to placing the patient in the Trende-lenberg position. In our experience this complication occurs in approx-imately 1–2% of patients during or immediately after flexible sigmo-idoscopy. It may also occur when a patient stands up rapidly, particu-larly following a difficult procedure. If response to Trendelenberg position is incomplete, intravenous fluids may be indicated for a brief period. Hypotension may also be the result of an arrhythmia, pulmonary embo-lism, or acute myocardial infarction, but other associated clinical fea-tures should be present to help detect these more ominous and fortu-nately rare events.

Electrocardiographic changes   Cardiographic monitoring has been performed during both rigid sigmoidoscopy and colonoscopy. ECG changes, including sinus tachycardia, bradycardia, ST segment changes, and ectopic beats, have been reported in up to 57% of patients under-going rigid sigmoidoscopy.[14] Sinus tachycardia was the most common rhythm disturbance followed by premature ventricular beats. The ectopic beats are more common in patients with underlying heart disease. All of the ECG changes in the study of 100 consecutive rigid sigmoidosco-pies occurred randomly throughout the procedure and were transient.[14]

In patients undergoing colonoscopy, continuous ECG monitoring has shown changes in 41%[1] and 65%[46] of patients in two series. As with sigmoidoscopy, sinus tachycardia and premature ventricular beats were the most common rhythm changes, occurring more frequently in patients with heart disease. Rare instances of cardiac arrest and acute myocardial infarction have occurred during colonoscopy.[40] Cardiac arrhythmias during colonoscopy may be related to many factors, including (1) stress of the procedure; (2) increased catecholamine response from anxiety; (3) effect of medication; or (4) hypovolemia from the bowel preparation. With flexible sigmoidoscopy, medications are usually not used, and the minimal bowel preparation should not result in hypovolemia. However, even flexible sigmoidoscopy may produce a certain amount of physical and psychological stress that may result in an arrhythmia, particularly in elderly patients with heart disease. A gentle technique, minimal air insufflation, and reassurance should minimize these cardiac risks. In selected patients with known, severe cardiac disease, ECG monitoring during the procedure is advisable. In all cases a nurse or assistant should observe the patient's pain response, color, respirations, pulse, and blood pressure at periodic intervals.

Bacteremia

Transient asymptomatic bacteremia has been reported in 9.5% of patients after rigid sigmoidoscopy.[22] While Norfleet et al.[32] and Rafoth et al.[36] found no bacteremia after colonoscopy, Pelican et al.[34] found an incidence of 27% when cultures were taken frequently during the first fifteen minutes of the procedure. Dickman et al.[11] noted a 4% incidence of bacteremia following colonoscopy. The organisms encountered in these studies represented the full range of colonic flora. It is likely that flexible sigmoidoscopy will also result in some incidence of bacteremia, since the procedure involves mechanical manipulation of the mucous membrances in an area with a large bacterial population. There have been two recent case reports of enterococcal endocarditis following both rigid sigmoidoscopy[37] and flexible sigmoidoscopy.[38] Although symptomatic bacteremia may be rare, it would seem advisable to:

- Thoroughly cleanse the flexible sigmoidoscope between procedures (see Chapter 2).
- Give antibiotic prophylaxis to granulocytopenic patients and patients with prosthetic heart valves, artificial joints, and those on hemodialysis who have arteriovenous shunts. The usual recommended regimen is ampicillin (1 g) and an aminoglycoside (gentamycin, 2 mg per kg) given intravenously about 30 minutes prior to the procedure and a second dose of each antibiotic six hours after the procedure.[38]

Table 9-4
Complications of Colonoscopic Polypectomy

Risk	Incidence*
Perforation	0.3–1.4%
Hemorrhage	0.7–2.5%
Cardiopulmonary	0.3%
Miscellaneous	0.1%
Total	1.0–4.0%

*See references 9,27,40.

COMPLICATIONS OF COLONOSCOPIC POLYPECTOMY

The major risks of colonoscopic polypectomy are perforation (0.3–1.4%) and hemorrhage (0.7–2.5%) (Table 9-4). It is likely that polypectomy performed via the flexible sigmoidoscope has similar risks to that of polypectomy at colonoscopy. Chapter 3 outlines the principles of electrosurgery and the correct polypectomy technique. Some common errors that may significantly increase risks for bleeding and perforation will be outlined.

It is important to recognize that the indications for polypectomy during flexible sigmoidoscopy are limited. When a polyp is found during a screening flexible sigmoidoscopy, there is a 25–40% incidence of proximal synchronous polyps and a 1–2% incidence of a synchronous cancer.[48] Further work-up including double-contrast barium enema and/or colonoscopy is generally indicated and polypectomy can be accomplished during colonoscopy. In addition, for a *screening* flexible sigmoidoscopy, the patient has generally had a limited bowel preparation and combustible colonic gases may be present. Furthermore, polypectomy is technically demanding and should not be performed by the novice endoscopist.

If a limited segment of bowel remains after subtotal colonic resection, it is reasonable to use the flexible sigmoidoscope as a colonoscope for diagnosis and polypectomy. Occasionally a polyp in a difficult location cannot be adequately snared during colonoscopy. With its short length and responsiveness to torque, the flexible sigmoidoscope may be preferred over the colonoscope. Finally, in a patient with a known sigmoid polyp and a high quality double-contrast barium enema, it may

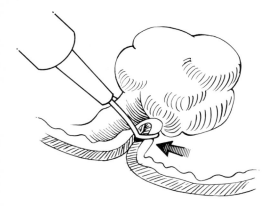

Figure 9-6. Improper snare placement. Bowel wall adjacent to pedicle of polyp (*arrow*) has been inadvertently snared.

be acceptable to remove the polyp via the flexible sigmoidoscope if colonoscopy is not available in the community.

Perforation

Perforation after polypectomy is uncommon (0.3–1.4%).[27,39] It usually presents with a major *free perforation* necessitating early laparotomy and colonic closure. Occasionally a *post-polypectomy coagulation syndrome*[48] may occur (see Table 9-3). This syndrome is a transmural burn of the colon without perforation and usually responds to conservative measures.

Several technical errors can lead to perforation. The adjacent bowel wall may be ensnared from an error in snare placement (Fig. 9-6). Too much electrocoagulation can result in a transmural burn or perforation. If the head of a polyp contacts the opposite wall during electrocoagulation, a burn on the opposite colonic wall may occur. If a sessile polyp is greater than 1.5 cm in diameter, it is safer to perform *piecemeal* removal in 2 or 3 sections (see Chapter 3). Piecemeal removal is technically difficult and should be performed only by very experienced operators. Mechanical or pneumatic pressures on the bowel wall, weakened by prior electrocoagulation, can lead to perforation. Failure to visualize the cauterization effect of a snare wire after looping a polyp may result in too little or too much coagulation.

Hemorrhage

Hemorrhage is the most common post-polypectomy complication (0.7–2.5%).[9,27,39] It may be minimal or massive and usually occurs within one to two hours of the procedure. However, one-third of patients may have delayed bleeding (1–21 days). Large pedunculated polyps (greater than 2.5 cm) are at greatest risk to bleed after resection since a large central blood vessel is usually present in their stalks.

Several technical errors can lead to hemorrhage. The electrocautery equipment may be faulty and therefore should always be checked before polypectomy. Rapid pull-through of the snare wire may result in *guillotining* the polyp, and thus slicing it off with the wire before completing electrocautery. To avoid this possibility the snare wire should not be fully closed until whitening occurs around the wire, signifying an electrocoagulative effect.

If bleeding does occur after polypectomy, several maneuvers may provide hemostasis. Adrenaline (5 ml of 1/1000) can be mixed with 50 cc of ice water and infused via a catheter onto the bleeding site. If a stalk is still present, it may be resnared and tightened. This tamponade effect may control hemorrhage. If bleeding continues, however, the stalk may be recauterized with the snare or electrocoagulation probe. If bleeding is massive, visceral angiography with selective intra-arterial infusion of pitressin may be helpful.[8] Occasionally, massive hemorrhage is uncontrollable and urgent surgery is indicated.

Explosions

An explosion from fulguration of colonic polyps during rigid sigmoidoscopy has been reported,[5] and there is a single report of a fatal explosion occurring during colonoscopic polypectomy.[3] Fortunately, this dramatic complication is exceedingly rare and the mechanisms and potential risk factors are well understood, making it totally preventable.

There are two combustible gases produced in the colon, hydrogen (H_2) and methane (CH_4). Hydrogen is produced by fermentation of unabsorbed carbohydrate by colonic bacteria, and methane is produced by bacterial metabolism unrelated to carbohydrate or other unabsorbed substrates.

Ragins et al. demonstrated combustible ranges of both H_2 and CH_4 in rectal gas samples from patients with unprepared colons.[35] However, after a standard preparation for colonoscopy, none of the patients had explosive mixtures in any part of the colon. Bond and Levitt also demonstrated a lack of combustible mixtures of colonic gases in patients following standard preparation for colonoscopy.[6] Preparation for flexible sigmoidoscopy usually involves only one or two Phospho-Soda enemas, and it is likely that some of these patients have combustible levels of H_2 and CH_4. To lessen the risk of an explosion from colonic gases, the patient undergoing polypectomy or any procedure where electrocautery is used, should have a full colon preparation. Other measures that can reduce the concentrations of combustible gases in the colon are air exchange with suction and insufflation during the procedure, and CO_2 insufflation. The use of CO_2 is probably unnecesary in an adequately prepared patient. The examination of the only report of an explosion during sigmoidoscopic fulguration of polyps reveals the patient's colon was inadequately prepared.[5] The only report of an explosion during colonoscopic polypectomy occurred in a patient who had been prepared with mannitol, a nonabsorbed carbohydrate which is fermented by bacteria to H_2.[3]

Explosion during flexible sigmoidoscopy should be preventable by observing the following rules (1) do not use any form of electrocoagulation if *only* the usual, limited bowel preparation is used; (2) if electrocoagulation is unavoidable, use CO_2 insufflation and/or exchange of air; (3) never use mannitol for bowel preparation; and (4) if polypectomy or other electrosurgery is planned, utilize a complete bowel preparation as for colonoscopy.

A good working knowledge of the electrocautery unit and snare equipment plus attention to detail should decrease the incidence of bleeding or perforation. Polypectomy should not be performed in situations (1) where significant abnormalities in blood coagulation exist; (2) after recent acetylsalicylic acid (aspirin) ingestion, which alters platelet function; and (3) with suspected invasive carcinoma in a polyp[41] (i.e., deformity, deep ulceration, discoloration, surface granularity, or disproportion in size of polyp head compared to the stalk).

Endoscopic polypectomy can be a rapid, relatively safe, and extremely rewarding procedure with an acceptable risk. Examiner knowledge and experience with close attention to details are very important in lessening the occurrence of complications.

REFERENCES

1. Alam M, Schuman BM, Duvernoy WFC, Madrago AC: Continuous elctrocardiographic monitoring during colonoscopy. Gastrointest Endosc 22:203–205, 1976
2. Berci G, Panish JF, Schapiro M, Corlin R: Complications of colonoscopy and polypectomy. Gastroenterology 67:584–585, 1974
3. Bigard MA, Gaucher P, Lassalle C: Fatal colonic explosion during colonoscopic polypectomy. Gastroenterology 77:1307–1310, 1979
4. Bohlman TW, Katon RM, Lipshutz G, et al.: Fiberoptic pansigmoidoscopy, an evaluation and comparison with rigid sigmoidoscopy. Gastroenterology 72:644–649, 1977
5. Bond JH, Levy M, Levitt MD: Explosion of hydrogen gas in the colon during proctosigmoidoscopy. Gastrointest Endosc 23:41–42, 1976

6. Bond JH, Levitt MD: Factors affecting the concentration of combustible gases in the colon during colonoscopy. Gastroenterology 68:1445–1448, 1975

7. Burt CA: Pneumatic rupture of the intestinal canal with experimental data showing the mechanism of perforation and the pressure required. Arch Surg 22:875–902, 1931

8. Carlyle DR, Goldstein HM: Angiographic management of bleeding following transcolonoscopic polypectomy. Dig Dis Sci 20:1196–1201, 1975

9. Cotton PB, Williams CB: Practical Gastroentestinal Endoscopy (2nd Ed.). London, Blackwell Scientific Publications, 1982, pp 142–154.

10. Crespi M, Casale V, Grassi A: Flexible sigmoidoscopy a potential advance in cancer control. Gastrointest Endosc. 24:291–292, 1978

11. Dickman MD, Farrell R, Higgs RH, et al.: Colonoscopy associated bacteremia. Surg Gynecol Obstet 142:173–176, 1976

12. Dagradi AE, Norris ME, Weingarten ZG: Delayed ("blow-out") perforation of sigmoid following diagnostic colonoscopy. Am J Gastroenterol 70:317–320, 1978

13. Echer MD, Goldstein M, Hoexter B, et al.: Benign pneumoperitoneum after fiberoptic colonoscopy. Gastroenterology 73:226–320, 1977

14. Fletcher GF, Earnest DL, Shuford WF, Wenger N: Electrocardiographic changes during routine sigmoidoscopy. Arch Intern Med 122:483–486, 1968

15. Geenan JE, Schmitt MG, Wu WC, Hogan WJ: Major complications of colonoscopy: Bleeding and perforation. Dig Dis Sci 20:231–235, 1975

16. Gilbert DA, Shaneyfelt SL, Mahler AK, et al.: The national ASGE colonoscopy surgery—Preliminary analysis of complications of colonoscopy. Gastrointest Endosc (Abstract) 29:191, 1983.

17. Hillman LC, Davies WA, Clarke AC: Fibersigmoidoscopy technique of choice? Med J Australia 1:548–549, 1980

18. Holt RW, Wherry DC: Why flexible fiberoptic sigmoidoscopy is important in the geriatric patient. Geriatrics 34:85–88, 1979

19. Johnson RA, Quan M, Rodney WM: Flexible sigmoidoscopy in primary care. The procedure and its potential. Postgrad Med 72:151–156, 1982

20. Katon RM, Melnyk CS: The pansigmoidoscope: One year's experience in a gastrointestinal diagnostic unit. J Clin Gastroenterol 1:41–45, 1979

21. Kozarek RA, Earnest DL, Silverstein ME, Smith RG: Air-pressure-induced colon injury during diagnostic colonoscopy. Gastroenterology 78:7–14, 1980

22. LeFrock JL, Ellis CA, Turchick JB, Weinstein L: Transient bacteremia associated with sigmoidoscopy. New Engl J Med 289:467–469, 1973

23. Leicester RJ, Hawley PR, Pollett WG, Nichols RJ: Flexible fiberoptic sigmoidoscopy as an outpatient procedure. Lancet 1:34–35, 1982

24. Lezak MB, Goldhamer M: Retroperitoneal emphysema after colonoscopy. Gastroenterology 66:118–120, 1974

25. Lipshutz GR, Katon RM, McCool MF, et al.: Flexible sigmoidoscopy as a screening procedure for neoplasia of the colon. Surg Gynecol Obstet 148:19–22, 1979

26. Livstone EM, Cohen GM, Trongale FJ, Touloukion MD: Diastatic serosal lacerations: An unrecognized complication of colonoscopy. Gastroenterology 67:1245–1247, 1974

27. Lobitz J, Katon RM: Handbook of gastrointestinal emergencies. Garden City, Medical Exam Publishing Co., 1982, pp 325–397.
28. Macrae FA, Tan KG, Williams CP: Toward safer colonoscopy: A report on the complications of 5000 diagnostic or therapeutic colonoscopies. Gut 24:376–383, 1983
29. Manier JW: Fiberoptic pansigmoidoscopy: An evaluation of its use in an office practice. Gastrointest Endosc 24:119–120, 1978
30. Marks G, Boggs W, Castro AF, et al.: Sigmoidoscopic examinations with rigid and flexible fiberoptic sigmoidoscopes in the surgeon's office: A comparative prospective study of effectiveness in 1,012 cases. Dis Colon Rectum 22:162–168, 1979
31. Meyer CT, McBride W. Goldblatt RS, et al.: Clinical experience with flexible sigmoidoscopy in asymptomatic and symptomatic patients. Yale J Biol Med 53:345–352, 1980
32. Norfleet RG, Mitchell PD, Mulholland DD, Philo, J: Does bacteremia follow colonoscopy? II. Results with blood cultures obtained 5, 10 and 15 minutes after colonoscopy. Gastrointest Endosc 23:31–32, 1976
33. O'Connor JJ: Flexible sigmoidoscopy: Is it of value? Am Surg 45:647–648, 1979
34. Pelican G, Hentges D, Butt J, et al.: Bacteremia during colonoscopy. Gastrointest Endosc 23:33–36, 1976
35. Ragins H, Shinya H, Wolff WI: The explosive potential of colonic gas during colonoscopic electrosurgical polypectomy. Surg Gynecol Obstet 138:554–556, 1974
36. Rafoth RJ, Sorenson RM, Bond JH: Bacteremia following colonoscopy. Gastrointest Endosc 22:32–33, 1975
37. Rigilono J, Mahopotra R, Barnhill J, et al.: Enterococcal endocarditis following sigmoidoscopy and mitral valve prolapse. Arch Intern Med 144:850–851, 1984
38. Rodriquez W, Levine JS: Enterococcal endocarditis following flexible sigmoidoscopy. West J Med 40:951–953, 1984
39. Rogers BH: Complications and hazards of colonoscopy, in Hunt RH & Waye JD (Eds.): Colonoscopy Techniques. Year Book Med Pub, 1981, pp. 237–264
40. Rogers BHG, Silvis SE, Nebel OT, et al.: Complications of flexible fiberopeptic colonoscopy and polypectomy. Gastrointest Endosc 22:73–76, 1975
41. Shinya H: One man's experience with 7386 polyps. Gastrointest Endosc 27:186–187, 1981
42. Sjogren RW, Johnson LF, Butler ML, et al.: Serosal laceration: A complication of intra-operative colonoscopy explained by transmucosal pressure gradients. Gastroenterology 24:239–242, 1978
43. Smith LL, Nivatvongs S: Complications in colonoscopy. Dis Colon Rectum 18:214–220, 1975
44. Spencer RJ, Wolff BG, Ready RN: Comparison of the rigid sigmoidoscope and the flexible sigmoidoscope in conjunction with colon x-ray for detection of lesions of the colon and rectum. Dis Colon Rectum 26:653–655, 1983

45. Traul DG, Davis CB, Pollock JC, Scudamore H: Flexible fiberoptic sigmo-idoscopy—The Monroe Clinic experience. Dis Colon Rectum 26:161–166, 1983
46. Vawter M, Ruiz R, Alaama A, et al.: Electrocardiographic monitoring during colonoscopy. Am J Gastroenterol 63:155–157, 1975
47. Vellacott KD, Hardcastle JD: An evaluation of flexible fiberoptic sigmoidos-copy. Brit Med J 283:1583–1586, 1981
48. Waye JD: The postpolypectomy coagulation syndrome. Gastrointest Endosc 27:184–186, 1981
49. Winawer SJ, Leidner SD, Boyle C, Kurtz RC: Comparison of flexible sig-moidoscopy with other diagnostic techniques in the diagnosis of rectocolon neoplasia. Dig Dis Sci 24:277–281, 1979
50. Winnan G, Berci G, Panish J, et al.: Superiority of the flexible to the rigid sigmoidoscope in routine proctosigmoidoscopy. N Eng J Med 302:1011–1012, 1980
51. Yassinger S, Midgley R, Cantor DS, et al.: Retroperitoneal emphysema after colonic polypectomy. West J Med 128:347–350, 1978

10

Screening For Colorectal Cancer and Polyps

Since the etiologic factors responsible for colorectal cancer are not known, prevention of disease is not yet possible and reliance must be placed on early detection utilizing screening techniques. Table 10-1 lists several general criteria of diseases amenable to screening and the reasons why colorectal cancer meets all of these criteria.[4,5,8] Colorectal cancer is more common than all other gastrointestinal malignancies combined, with approximately 150,000 new cases predicted per year in the United States. Most physicians and a large segment of the public at risk are knowledgeable about colon cancer, but screening techniques are only variably implemented in routine practice. This chapter will deal mainly with early detection of colorectal cancer and its precursor lesion, the adenomatous polyp, by use of screening techniques such as fecal occult blood tests, digital rectal examination and flexible sigmoidoscopy.

Screening studies have demonstrated that colon cancer detected during an asymptomatic phase is usually an early lesion,[10,19,31] and that the expected 5-year survival is nearly twice the 40% survival rate for patients with symptomatic lesions. An important question regarding screening is whether the diagnostic services necessary for complete work-up after a positive screening test are available in every community. It is likely that some communities would have their current radiologic and gastroenterologic manpower severely taxed if mass screening were applied. For example, in a community of 60,000 people, perhaps 20,000 individuals will be over 50 years of age and eligible for screening. If 5% have a positive fecal occult blood test, then 1000 double-contrast barium enemas and/or colonoscopies are indicated. Based on current statistics, approximately 100 or so individuals from this population base will have

Table 10-1
Colon Cancer: A Disease Amenable to Screening

General Disease Criteria	Fulfillment of Criteria by Colon Cancer
Relatively common	~150,000 new cases/yr. in U.S. (est. for 1985)
Serious consequences	40% 5-yr. survival and 75,000 deaths/yr. in U.S.
Recognized as a problem by physicians and patients	Yes
Asymptomatic phase during which screening tests can detect disease	Yes, with detection by fecal occult blood testing and/or flexible sigmoidoscopy
Available health services adequate for diagnostic follow-up of positive screening tests	Double-contrast barium enema and colonoscopy or flexible sigmoidoscopy widely available
Therapy during asymptomatic phase will favorably alter the natural history	5-yr. survival after surgical resection: 40% for symptomatic and 70–80% for asymptomatic patients
Effective therapy	Surgical resection of cancer and/or colonoscopic polypectomy effective and widely available

asymptomatic colorectal cancer, most of who could be readily treated by available surgeons. This example demonstrates that full implementation of screening techniques reviewed in this chapter will have a major impact on physician manpower and medical economics.

COLORECTAL CANCER

A few basic concepts regarding colorectal cancer, including Dukes' classification, polyp–cancer sequence, and risk factors for colon cancer, will be briefly reviewed before addressing the topic of screening.

Dukes' Classification

Although many variations have been proposed, the standard Dukes' classification remains a useful index of prognosis of colorectal cancer[6] (Table 10-2). When newly diagnosed patients with colorectal cancer are

Table 10-2
Dukes' Classification of Colorectal Cancer*

Stage	Definition	5-Year Survival (%)
Dukes' A	Cancer limited to mucosa	95
Dukes' B	Cancer extending to serosa	65
Dukes' C	Cancer involving lymph nodes	30
Dukes' D	Distant metastases	<5

*Reference 6.

divided into asymptomatic and symptomatic groups, asymptomatic individuals are far more likely to have a favorable Dukes' status (Table 10-3). Approximately 75–85% of asymptomatic but only 40% of symptomatic patients will have an early Dukes' A or B stage with the better 5-year survivals as outlined in Table 10-2. Unfortunately, most patients with colorectal cancer are not diagnosed until they reach a symptomatic stage characterized by abdominal pain, bloody stools, tenesmus, altered bowel habits, and/or anemia. Widespread screening has the potential to reverse this current major medical problem and diagnose the majority of patients in an earlier asymptomatic phase of their cancer or even before cancer evolves from a premalignant polyp.

Polyp-Cancer Sequence

This concept was formerly very controversial. There is now little doubt that most colorectal cancers (~95%) arise from colorectal adenomatous polyps.[7,9,17] Several lines of evidence support this thesis. Both

Table 10-3
Distribution of Newly Diagnosed Patients with Colorectal Cancer by Dukes' Classification*

Stage	Asymptomatic (%)	Symptomatic (%)
Dukes' A	50	10
Dukes' B	25	30
Dukes' C	20	40
Dukes' D	5	20

*References 18,30.

polyps and cancer have a similar distribution in the colon, with 65–70% of both lesions located in the left colon. Furthermore, approximately 10% of resected polyps contain an area of adenocarcinoma, directly supporting a polyp–cancer sequence. The larger the polyp, the greater the likelihood it has of harboring cancer (<1 cm = 1%; 1–2 cm = 10%; >2 cm = 25–40%). This observation suggests that malignant degeneration occurs as polyps grow in size. Moreover, minute colon cancers are extremely rare, even in autopsy series, suggesting that colon cancer does not begin de novo but arises from pre-existing colorectal polyps. Further evidence to support the polyp-cancer sequence is demonstated by the inherited disorder of familiar polyposis, where the bowel is carpeted with thousands of adenomatous polyps and the condition carries an extreme risk for the development of colorectal cancer. Finally, diagnosis and sigmoidoscopic removal of rectal polyps was shown to decrease the subsequent incidence of rectal cancer by 85%.[4]

With these facts in mind, it is undoubtedly important to screen not only for early colorectal cancer but also for its precursor lesion, the adenomatous polyp. The progression from polyp to cancer is slow, averaging 5–15 years.[31] Therefore, screening, detection, and colonoscopic removal of polyps should be very effective in preventing a colorectal malignancy.

Risk Factors for Colorectal Cancer

Once the importance of detecting both asymptomatic colon cancer and adenomatous polyps is appreciated, the population at risk needs to be defined. The degree of risk will determine which screening test(s) should be used, at what age they should be applied, and how often the tests will be necessary.[8,20]

Table 10-4 lists the recognized risk factors for colorectal cancer and the degree of risk for each group. Later in the chapter the application of screening techniques for each risk level is discussed. In the following section, the available screening procedures will be reviewed.

SCREENING TESTS FOR COLORECTAL CANCER

Fecal Occult Blood Tests

The fecal occult blood tests in widespread use between 1945 and 1967 included the "bench" guaiac test, benzidine test, and the Hematest (Orthotolidine method). These tests were not standardized, and there was a high percentage of false positive and false negative results.[21] In

Table 10-4.
Risk Factors for Colorectal Cancer and Polyps*

Average Risk	High Risk (1.5–5-fold)	Very High Risk (>10-fold)	Extreme Risk (>100-fold)
Age > 40–50 years	Prior colonic polypectomy	Ulcerative colitis	Familial polyposis coli
	Prior colonic cancer resection	• Universal—risk begins after 8–10 years of disease	Gardner's syndrome
	Prior cancer of breast or uterus	• Left-sided—risk begins after 20 years of disease	Family history of either of above (autosomal dominant)
	Multiple juvenile polyposis		
	Crohn's colitis	Family cancer syndrome	
	Peutz-Jeghers syndrome		
	Dermal skin tags	Site-specific colon cancer (right colon)	
	Family history of colon cancer or polyps		

*Reference 5,8.

1967 Greegor reintroduced the guaiac test in a modified and standardized form consisting of filter paper slides impregnated with guaiac.[11] The stool was smeared on the impregnated paper and then tested with a reagent of hydrogen peroxide in denatured alcohol. This test, initially manufactured as Hemoccult*, and later modified to Hemoccult II, has been widely used in the U.S. and elsewhere (Fig. 10-1). The application of Hemoccult II for screening has also been standardized over recent years. Stool is collected while ingesting a high fiber diet with no rare red meat and no raw fruits and vegetables containing large amounts of peroxidase. The diet should begin two days prior to testing and should be continued during the 3-day test period. Iron and nonsteroidal anti-inflammatory drugs should be precluded. Stools are collected on three consecutive days, and two samples are tested from each stool for a total of six slides. Table 10-5 summarizes the clinical data obtained with this test in several screening studies.[10,12,30,31]

---

*Hemoccult and Hemoccult II are registered trademarks of SmithKline Diagnostics, Inc.

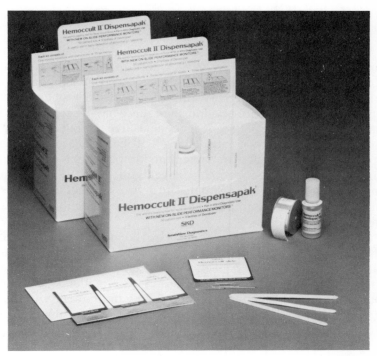

Figure 10-1. Hemoccult II Dispensapak with slides, applicator sticks, developer, and mailing envelopes. (Photograph supplied courtesy of SmithKline Diagnostics, Inc., Sunnyvale, California.)

Table 10-5
Results of Fecal Occult Blood Testing in an Asymptomatic Population
Over 50 Years of Age*

Result	Reported Range (%)
Patient compliance	15–80
Incidence of positive slides	3–5
Predictive value of a positive slide for colorectal neoplasia	40–50
Stage Dukes' A or B cancers	70–85
False-positive rate	1.5–2.5
False-negative rate for cancer	10–30
False-negative rate for adenomas	65–75

$\nearrow$ ¼ cancer

$\searrow$ ¾ adenomatous polyps

*References 8,10,12,31.

Patient compliance with fecal occult blood testing ranges from 15% in an unmotivated population to 80% in a private practice situation. The incidence of positive slides is 3–5% in asymptomatic patients over the age of 50. The predictive value of a positive test for colorectal neoplasia is 40–50%, with one-fourth of these having colon cancer and three-fourths harboring polyps. Even one positive test out of six demands a thorough diagnostic workup, which will be discussed later in this chapter. Cancers detected in asymptomatic patients by Hemoccult II testing generally have a favorable stage, with Dukes' A and B lesions accounting for 70–85% of the total. The 5-year survival in these asymptomatic individuals should thus be better than patients having symptomatic lesions.

Screening for colorectal neoplasia by Hemoccult II has a significant false positive and false negative rate (Table 10-5). Although the false positive rate is low at 1.5–2.5% of subjects screened, this percentage accounts for half of all positive slides (3–5% incidence). When large populations are subjected to screening, many individuals will therefore undergo unnecessary and costly procedures such as double-contrast barium enema and colonoscopy. Plant, bacterial, and animal (meat) peroxidases account for some of the false positive tests and other colonic lesions (diverticuli, arteriovenous malformations, etc.) or upper gastrointestinal lesions (peptic ulcer, gastric cancer, etc.) make up the remainder. Iron or nonsteroidal anti-inflammatory drugs can also pro-

Table 10-6
Fecal Occult Blood Tests Available in the United States

Manufacturer	Product
SmithKline Diagnostics, Inc. Sunnyvale, CA	Hemoccult II
Helena Laboratories Beaumont, TX	Colo Screen
Miles Laboratories Elkhart, IN	Hema-Chek
Gamma Diagnostic Houston, TX	Fe-Cult Plus

duce false positive tests. Finally, rehydration of the Hemoccult II slide makes the test overly sensitive and will increase the false positive results.

Hemoccult II testing also has a significant false negative rate that is greater for colonic polyps than for cancer. Potential reasons for false negative tests include (1) absent, minimal, or intermittent bleeding from nonulcerated tumors or small polyps; (2) inhomogenous mixture of blood in the stool; (3) vitamin C ingestion (interferes with peroxidase test); (4) delay in adding the reagent to the slide (positivity decays slightly when tested more than five days from time of smear); or (5) failure to follow a high bulk diet. The false negative rate of fecal occult blood tests for colon cancer ranges from 10–30% and correlates with the absence of ulceration of the tumor.[12] Rehydration of slides may increase the sensitivity for colorectal cancer,[16] but is generally not employed since it also increases the false positive rate. Fecal occult blood testing is generally too insensitive for reliable detection of colonic polyps, since the false negative rate is as high as 65–75%. [3,15,30] This rate varies with adenoma size, however, and lesions over 2 cm may give positive Hemoccult tests in 75% of patients while lesions below 1 cm yield positive tests in only 7%.[14]

In addition to Hemoccult II, several other fecal occult blood tests are available in the United States and all employ guaiac impregnated paper (Table 10-6). In 1984 Menley & James Laboratories, a SmithKline Bockman Company, introduced the Hemoccult Home Test, which is available over-the-counter in pharmacies. More specific and sensitive fecal occult blood tests are being evaluated. Using a specific anti-human hemoglobin, Turunen et al. reported a qualitative immunological test.[26] The results were impressive in that 29 of 30 patients with known colorectal cancer had a positive test with an overall false negative rate of only 3%. This test is relatively time consuming and expensive, and not yet applicable for mass screening. Schwartz et al.[23] described the HemoQuant test, a specific quantitative test of hemoglobin in feces. This test is also specific and sensitive, but is too time consuming for widespread application.

Sigmoidoscopy

The yield of rigid sigmoidoscopy has been evaluated in numerous screening studies of asymptomatic patients for colorectal neoplasia. Adenomatous polyps are found in approximately 5–10% of subjects, while carcinomas are noted in only 0.1–0.2% of individuals.[15,26] Ward et al.[27] felt that the cost to detect colorectal cancer by routine sigmoidoscopy in an asymptomatic population would be excessive. In 1966 Moertel et al.[17] challenged the role of colorectal screening for neoplasia with sigmoidoscopy, since the yield of carcinoma was so low. He doubted the value of finding or removing polyps since the polyp–cancer sequence was questioned at that time. Within 10 years, however, it became generally accepted that perhaps 95% of all colon cancers do in fact arise from adenomatous polyps.[18] In a landmark study, Gilbertsen[9] performed annual rigid sigmoidoscopy in more than 18,000 patients over a 25-year period. He removed all polypoid lesions within the reach of the sigmoidoscope. Participants in this study were noted to have an 85% decrease in the anticipated rate of adenocarcinoma of the rectosigmoid area, thus strongly supporting effective prevention of cancer by polyp removal. In a screening program at the Strang Clinic, 50 asymptomatic patients with rectal cancer were detected with rigid sigmoidoscopy, and had an impressive 90% 5-year survival.[13] Since nearly 75% of polyps and 10–30% of cancers are not diagnosed by fecal occult blood studies, sigmoidoscopy should be included with fecal occult blood testing in screening programs for colorectal neoplasia.

The former belief that 65–70% of polypoid lesions were within reach of the rigid sigmoidoscope is no longer tenable. In the past two decades, there has been a dramatic change in the site of polyp and cancer distribution, with more proximal sigmoid lesions and fewer rectal lesions.[24] At best only 30–40% of all colonic neoplastic lesions can now be found with the rigid instrument. In the late 1970's flexible sigmoidoscopes with lengths of 35 cm and 60 cm became available. These instruments were shown to detect at least twice as many polypoid lesions as the rigid instrument.[2,34] Lipshutz et al.[15] noted a 12% incidence of adenomatous polyps in asymptomatic males over the age of 50 years when screened with a 60-cm instrument. Only 18% of the polyps detected were below 20 cm and therefore within the average rigid sigmoidoscopic range. Wherry[28] found a 12.5% incidence of adenomatous polyps during screening examinations in asymptomatic patients over 50 years of age. Only 50% were within the 25-cm range from the anal verge.

The use of the 25-cm rigid sigmoidoscope thus appears to have limited effectiveness in screening for colorectal neoplasia. Over the next several years there will likely be a gradual switch from routine use of rigid to flexible sigmoidoscopy. In order for this evolution to occur, large numbers of primary care physicians and perhaps paramedical personnel will need to be trained in flexible sigmoidoscopy.

Digital Rectal Examination

This is a very simple and safe means of evaluating the anal canal and distal rectum. Tumors within 7–8 cm of the anal verge can usually be palpated. The American Cancer Society recommends digital rectal examination yearly, beginning at age 40.

Application of Screening Techniques

How often should the general population at average risk for colorectal neoplasia undergo screening fecal occult blood testing and sigmoidoscopy? At what age should screening be initiated?

The risk for colorectal cancer increases at age 40 and rises even more sharply after age 50. Therefore, screening techniques should be applied to the average risk population beginning at age 40–50 (Table 10-7). The fecal occult blood test is simple and inexpensive and can detect lesions that bleed from any part of the gastrointestinal tract. It should probably be performed yearly in patients over 40 years of age.

It is now recognized that the polyp-to-cancer transformation is slow and usually occurs over several years. In addition, colon cancer is generally slow growing, taking at least 5 years to grow from 1–5 cm.[7] It is thus unnecessary to perform yearly sigmoidoscopy as was once recommended. In 1980 the American Cancer Society recommended that the general population undergo sigmoidoscopy every 3–5 years after 2 yearly negative exams in patients 50 years of age or greater.[1]

Screening techniques are applied earlier and at different intervals in patients with a higher risk for colorectal cancer (Table 10-7). In some of these high risk categories, screening tests may not be sufficient and more elaborate diagnostic tests such as double-contrast barium enema and/or colonoscopy may be recommended at regular intervals.

Table 10-7
Recommendations for Screening Normal and High-Risk Individuals for Colorectal Neoplasia[‡]

Risk	Age (yr)	Test(s)
Average	≥40	Annual digital rectal examination and fecal occult blood test
	≥50	Above protocol plus sigmoidoscopy* q3–5 yr after two negative annual sigmoidoscopies
High (1.5–5 × normal) History of genital or breast cancer Family history of colorectal polyps or cancer Presence of skin tags	35–40	Annual fecal occult blood test and sigmoidoscopy* q3–5 yr
Prior resection of colon cancer Prior polypectomy	all ages	Colonoscopy 1 year after procedure, thereafter annual fecal occult blood test and colonoscopy[†] q3–5 yr
Very High (10 × normal) Family cancer syndrome Site-specific colon cancer	20	Annual fecal occult blood test and colonoscopy[†] q3–5 yr
Chronic ulcerative colitis • Universal disease • Left-sided disease	8–10 yr after onset 15–20 yr after onset	Annual colonoscopy with multiple biopsies; total colectomy if severe dyplasia found
Extreme Risk (>100 × normal) 1st degree relative with multiple adenomatous polyposis	Teens	Sigmoidoscopy q6 months until age 40; subtotal or total colectomy if positive for multiple polyposis. Screening enzyme test in development

*Either 35-cm or 60-cm flexible sigmoidoscopy preferred to rigid sigmoidoscopy.
[†]Colonoscopy is preferred, but double-contrast barium enema plus flexible sigmoidoscopy may be substituted.
[‡]Reference number 22, 33.

EVALUATION OF THE PATIENT WITH A POSITIVE SCREENING TEST

Nearly 50% of patients with a positive fecal occult blood test harbor a polyp or cancer in the colon. When sigmoidoscopy reveals a polyp, 25–40% of these patients harbor additional, proximal polypoid lesions.[32] Therefore, a complete colonic examination is in order when either of these screening tests is positive.

Several techniques are available to evaluate the colon. The single contrast barium enema has been employed for years but may miss as many as 42% of all polypoid lesions in the colon.[35] This technique should probably no longer be used for detection of neoplasia in asymptomatic patients with positive screening tests. Although slightly more time-consuming and uncomfortable than the standard barium enema, double-contrast barium enema is much more sensitive for the diagnosis of polypoid lesions. Williams et al.[29] detected 98% of all polyps over 1 cm and 78% of all polyps under 1 cm by double-contrast barium enema. With standard barium enema, they found only 77% of polyps over 1 cm, and only 18% of those under 1 cm.

Total colonoscopy, performed with modern fiberscopes by well-trained individuals, allows visualization to the cecum in over 90% of cases.[29,35] The procedure, however, requires sedation, 30–45 minutes to perform in most cases, and a small but definite risk of perforation (~1/500). Colonoscopy is extremely accurate but may miss between 5 and 10% of colonic lesions. Missed lesions are either in proximal areas not reached by examination or hidden behind haustral folds.[14] Since most lesions missed by double-contrast barium enema are in the sigmoid colon,[25,35] colonoscopy may be complementary to double-contrast barium enema by providing thorough visualization of this part of the colon. In addition, most polypoid lesions can safely be removed during colonoscopy.

Although full colonoscopy plus double-contrast barium enema is the "gold standard" of colonic evaluation, some communities may not have ready access to colonoscopy. Since 60-cm flexible sigmoidoscopy will visualize the sigmoid colon well, it may be used to complement the double-contrast barium enema. Winawer[34] studied 81 Hemoccult positive patients with this combination of tests and found all 8 cancers and 85% of polyps seen by colonoscopy. Table 10-8 represents our estimate of the diagnostic accuracy of various combinations of techniques used to evaluate patients with a positive fecal occult blood test. It may be that colonoscopy alone, performed by a competent endoscopist, may be justified as the initial diagnostic examination following a positive screening test. Colonoscopy, if completed to the cecum, is very accurate, and also allows a polypectomy to be performed. If colonoscopy is not complete, then double-contrast barium enema can be performed.

Table 10-8
Estimated Percentage of Colorectal Neoplastic Lesions Detected by
Various Diagnostic Tests

Diagnostic Test(s)	Polyps (%)	Cancer (%)
Rigid sigmoidoscopy and single-contrast BE*	50–60	75–85
Flexible sigmoidoscopy (60-cm) and double-contrast BE	80–90	90–95
Colonoscopy	90–95	95
Colonoscopy and double-contrast BE	95–100	98–100

*BE = barium enema.

This topic is in a state of flux, and several acceptable alternatives are available for evaluation of the patient with a positive screening test. If a complete colon evaluation proves negative, evaluation of the upper GI tract should be performed.

Table 10-7 summarizes the recommended approach to screening the normal population and those individuals with higher risk for colorectal neoplasia. These suggestions are general and may not fit every situation. Both screening and diagnostic testing should be tailored to each patient. For instance, a patient who has seven or eight adenomatous polyps scattered throughout the colon probably has a much higher risk of recurrent lesions than a patient with a single adenoma and should probably be re-evaluated at shorter intervals.

Despite advances in both screening and diagnostic tests, a formidable task awaits physicians in the coming years. Effective screening of large numbers of patients requires increased awareness of the problem by both patients and physicians, regular application of fecal occult blood tests, greater use of flexible sigmoidoscopy, and appropriate referral for diagnostic techniques, such as double contrast barium enema and colonoscopy. The costs incurred by full implementation of screening techniques will no doubt be great, but detection and removal of polyps and early carcinoma should significantly reduce the morbidity and mortality of patients with colorectal neoplasia.

REFERENCES

1. American Cancer Society: Cancer of the colon and rectum. CA 30:208–215, 1980.
2. Bohlman T, Katon RM, Lipshutz G, et al.: Fiberoptic pansigmoidoscopy— an evaluation and comparison with rigid sigmoidoscopy. Gastroenterology 72:644–649, 1977.

3. Chapius PH, Goulston KJ, Pheils MT: Screeing of patients after surgery for colorectal carcinoma. Med J Aust 1:538–540, 1980.
4. Cole P, Morrison AS: Basic issues in population screening for cancer. J Natl Cancer Institute 64:1263–1273, 1980.
5. Diehl AK: Screening for colorectal cancer. J Fam Pract 12:625–632, 1981.
6. Dukes CE: The classification of cancer of the rectum. J Pathol Bacteriol 35:323–332, 1932.
7. Ekelind G, Lindstrüm C, Rosengren JE: Appearance and growth of early carcinomas of the colon-rectum. Acta Radiol 15:670–679, 1974.
8. Fath RB, Winawer SJ: Early diagnosis of colorectal cancer. Ann Rev Med 34:501–517, 1983.
9. Gilbertsen VA: Proctosigmoidoscopy and polypectomy in reducing the incidence of rectal cancer. Cancer 34:936–939, 1974.
10. Gilbertsen VA, McHugh R, Schuman L, et al.: The earlier detection of colorectal cancer: A preliminary report of the results of the occult blood study. Cancer 45:2899–2901, 1980.
11. Greegor DH: Diagnosis of large bowel cancer in the asymptomatic patient. JAMA 201:943–945, 1967.
12. Griffith CDM, Turner DJ, Saunders JH: False-negative results of hemoccult test in colorectal cancer. Brit Med J 283:472, 1981.
13. Hertz RL, Deddish MR, Day E: Value of periodic examination in detecting cancer of the rectum and colon. Postgrad Med 27:290–294, 1960.
14. Laufer I, Smith NCW, Mullens JE: The radiological demonstration of colorectal polyps undetected by endoscopy. Gastroenterology 70:167–170, 1976.
15. Lipshutz G, Katon RM, McCool M, et al.: Flexible sigmoidoscopy as a screening procedure for neoplasia of the colon. Surg, Gynec Obstet 148:19–22, 1979.
16. Macrae FA, St. John DJB: Relationship between patterns of bleeding and hemoccult sensitivity in patients with colorectal cancer or adenomas. Gastroenterology 82:891–898, 1982.
17. Moertel CG, Hill JR, Dockerty MB: The routine proctoscopic examination: A second look. Mayo Clin Proc 41:368–372, 1966.
18. Morson B: The polyp-cancer sequence in the large bowel. Proc Roy Soc Med 67:451–457, 1974.
19. Nivatvongs S, Gilbertsen VA, Goldberg SM, et al.: Distribution of large-bowel cancers detected by occult blood test in asymptomatic patients. Dis Colon Rectum 25:420–421, 1982.
20. Nostrant TT, Wilson JAP: How good is screening for colorectal cancer? Postgrad Med 73:131–139, 1983.
21. Ostrow JD, Mulvaney CA, Hansel JR, Rhodes RS: Sensitivity and reproductibility of chemical tests for fecal occult blood with an emphasis on false-positive reactions. Dig Dis Sci 18:930–940, 1973.
22. Riddell RH, Goldman H, Ronsohoff DF, et al.: Dysplasia in inflammatory bowel disease: Standardized classification with provisional clinical application. Human Pathol 14:931–938, 1983.
23. Schwartz S, Dahl J, Ellefson M, Ahlquist D: The "Hemo-Quant" test: A specific and quantitative determination of heme (hemoglobin) in feces and other materials. Clin Chem 29:2061–2067, 1983.

24. Snyder DN, Hesten JF, Meigs JW, Flannery JT: Changes in site distribution of colorectal carcinoma in Connecticutt, 1940–1973. Dig Dis Sci 22:791–797, 1977.
25. Thoeni RF, Menuck L: Comparison of barium enema and colonoscopy in the detection of small colonic polyps. Radiology 124:631–635, 1977.
26. Turunen MJ, Liewendahl K, Partanen P, Adlercreutz H: Immunological detection of faecal occult blood in colorectal cancer. Br J Cancer 49:141–148, 1984.
27. Ward KM, Bourdages R, Beck IT: A cost accounting of routine sigmoidoscopic examinations. CMA Journal 3:676–677, 1974.
28. Wherry DC: Screening for colorectal neoplasia in asymptomatic patients using flexible fiberoptic sigmoidoscopy. Dis Colon Rectum 24:521–522, 1981.
29. Williams CB, Hunt RH, Loose H, et al.: Colonoscopy in the management of colon polyps. Brit J Surg 61:673–682, 1974.
30. Winawer SJ, Fleischer M, Baldwin M, Sherlock P: Current status of fecal occult blood testing in screening for colorectal cancer. CA 32:101–112, 1982.
31. Winawer SJ, Andrews M, Flehinger B, et al.: Progress report on controlled trial of fecal occult blood testing for the detection of colorectal neoplasia. Cancer 45:2959–2964, 1980.
32. Winawer SJ, Fleischer M, Sherlock P: Sensitivity of fecal occult blood testing for adenomas. Gastroenterology 83:1136–ll37, 1982.
33. Winawer SJ, Sherlock P: Malignant neoplasms of the small and large intestine, in Sleisenger MH and Fordtran JS (Eds). Gastrointestinal Disease. Philadelphia, W.B. Saunders Co., 1983, pp 1220–1249.
34. Winawer SJ, Leidner SD, Boyle C, Kurtz RC: Comparison of flexible sigmoidoscopy with other diagnostic techniques in the diagnosis of rectocolon neoplasia. Dig Dis Sci 24:277–281, 1979.
35. Wolff WI, Shinya H, Geffen A, et al.: Comparison of colonoscopy and the contrast enema in 500 patients with colorectal disease. Am J Surg 129:181–186, 1975.

11

Diseases of the Rectosigmoid Colon

Careful inspection of the colonic mucosa during sigmoidoscopy is often the single most important step leading to the diagnosis of rectosigmoid diseases. The final diagnosis, however, is usually substantiated only after detailed history and physical examination is combined with appropriate use of ancillary tests, such as stool examination for parasites and culture for enteric pathogens, serologic tests, colonic mucosal biopsy, or barium enema x-ray. Some colonic diseases, such as ulcerative colitis or ischemic colitis, are diagnosed on the basis of typical sigmoidoscopic findings combined with compatible clinical, laboratory, and radiologic features and exclusion of infectious processes. In these diseases, accurate visual interpretation of the abnormal colonic mucosa has major diagnostic significance.

The purpose of this chapter is to review by brief description and endoscopic pictorial display the general characteristics of normal and abnormal mucosa and the typical sigmoidoscopic abnormalities seen in various diseases involving the rectosigmoid colon.

NORMAL RECTAL AND COLONIC MUCOSA

The normal rectal mucosa is smooth and glistening with a pale salmon-pink color (Fig. 11-1). Light from the sigmoidoscope is reflected uniformly from a broad area of mucosa. Branching submucosal blood vessels are easily visible as a reddish and bluish network seen through the normal mucosa and are most prominent in the rectum. The rectosigmoid colon is easily distensible with air, and the edges of the rectal valves are sharp. The most distal rectum can be inspected by retroflexion of the sigmoidoscope tip (Fig. 11-2). Internal hemorrhoids may be seen by this maneuver or during slow withdrawal of the instrument through the anus (Fig. 11-3).

Two variations from normal may be seen during flexible sigmoidoscopy and are worthy of comment. Some patients, many who have the diagnosis of irritable bowel syndrome, exhibit marked spasm of the sigmoid colon and experience severe pain during insertion of the sigmoidoscope. The irritable bowel syndrome is a very common disorder characterized by a wide variety of symptoms, of which the most characteristic are lower abdominal cramping pain and alteration of bowel habits with constipation and/or diarrhea.[16,29] A number of colonic motility abnormalities have been demonstrated both at rest and after stimulation by diet, hormones, or colonic distention with air.[16,29] These physiologic studies validate the common clinical observation that patients with irritable bowel syndrome often have prominent spasm of the sigmoid colon making full insertion of the sigmoidoscope difficult or impossible.

A second variation from normal found during flexible sigmoidoscopy in somewhat more than half of children and young adults is a slightly nodular colonic mucosa.[23] These nodules are smooth and round with occasional central umbilication, yellowish-white in color, and only 1–2 mm in diameter. Biopsy studies have demonstrated that they represent prominent mucosal lymph follicles, which probably develop in response to nonspecific stimuli. The younger the patient, the more likely that these nodules will be visualized.

MUCOSAL ABNORMALITIES OF THE RECTOSIGMOID COLON

A brief description of the general mucosal changes that occur in diseases of the rectosigmoid colon will be reviewed. Although some mucosal changes are characteristic of certain diseases, such as diffuse granularity and friability in ulcerative colitis or pseudomembranes in antibiotic-associated colitis, other mucosal abnormalities are nonspecific and found in numerous rectosigmoid diseases.

Edema and Erythema

Edema and erythema often accompany one another and are caused by increased interstitial fluid and inflammation within the submucosal space. As a result of these processes, the normal fine network of branching blood vessels is no longer seen through the mucosa. The normally smooth and glistening mucosa becomes irregular in height and loses its glistening appearance. The usually broad and uniform reflection of light from the sigmoidoscope is replaced by scattered multiple highlights. Edema and erythema are characteristic early findings in many forms of colitis, such as ulcerative colitis, but also are nonspecific mucosal changes that may result from diarrhea of any cause or from enema preparation prior to sigmoidoscopy.

Granularity

Granularity is a mucosal characteristic that develops with progressive inflammation of the submucosa. The term granularity is applied to an uneven mucosal surface that reflects irregular scattered pinpoints of light. Since much of the reflected light is lost, the mucosa takes on the appearance of a dry rather than moist surface. As the pathologic process advances, the granularity becomes more prominent and irregular with a change in appearance from *fine granularity* to *coarse granularity*. Associated with more severe granularity is the loss of sharpness of the rectal valves, which become blunted. These more advanced changes usually imply a chronic disease process.

Friability

Friability is closely associated with granularity, but represents a further abnormality of the mucosal surface. The normal colonic mucosa will not bleed when gently wiped with a cotton swab or lightly rubbed with the sigmoidoscope. By contrast, the mucosal surface in active ulcerative colitis bleeds easily when rubbed by the endoscope because the diseased mucosa has increased vascularity and diffuse erosions. In more advanced stages of colitis, the colonic mucosa may spontaneously ooze blood, so-called spontaneous friability. The mucosal characteristic of friability accounts for the rectal bleeding that often accompanies ulcerative colitis and other types of colitis.

Ulceration

A number of different types of ulceration may develop in the colonic mucosa. In ulcerative colitis, diffuse erosions and ulcerations are present but not often identified as discrete ulcers because of their superficial and uniform distribution. In Crohn's disease, however, ulcerations characteristically occur in areas of grossly normal mucosa. These ulcers may be punched out, linear, or serpiginous and may be deep or superficial and aphthous in character. Most discrete ulcers are surrounded by a narrow rim of erythema. Discrete ulcers may also be seen in amebic colitis, ischemic colitis, and as an isolated phenomenon in an otherwise normal colon (solitary ulcer of the rectum).

Mucus, Pus, and Exudate

Clear, white mucoid material is occasionally seen in the colonic lumen but is not adherent to the rectal or colonic mucosa. This finding is nonspecific and may occur as part of the irritable bowel syndrome or from nonspecific stimuli such as enemas. Pus and exudate are somewhat interchangeable terms that refer to yellow mucus that is more tenacious and is adherent to the wall of the colon. Exudate is commonly seen within the crater of larger ulcers and also found diffusely in miscellaneous types of colitis.

Pseudomembranes

Pseudomembranes are characteristic of pseudomembranous colitis, which is most often associated with antibiotic usage (antibiotic-associated colitis). Elevated yellowish-white plaques of variable size from a few mm to several cm are seen in the involved colon. Rarely, a complete pseudomembrane may overlie the mucosa. The mucosa between the pseudomembranous plaques is normal or shows only mild edema and erythema. Histologically, the pseudomembrane is composed of mucus, fibrin, and inflammatory cells overlying an area of mucosal ulceration.

Mass Lesions

A number of mass lesions may project into the colonic lumen. These lesions should be inspected carefully and described in detail with particular attention to features such as size, location, and overlying mucosa. Polyps can be characterized as either sessile or pedunculated. This determination may sometimes be assisted by the placement of biopsy forceps through the sigmoidoscope and manipulation of the head of the polyp. The morphology of the overlying mucosa should be compared to that of the surrounding normal mucosa. Adenocarcinomas may appear as polypoid tumors, bulky masses of friable tissue, or growths with a central crater and hard edges. Submucosal lesions such as lipomas and leiomyomas have an intact overlying mucosa similar to that of the surrounding mucosa. In severe forms of colitis, pseudopolyps may be seen. These lesions are projections of tissue composed of normal mucosa or granulation tissue that project from the mucosa like multiple fingers or can be large and sessile resembling an adenocarcinoma. On occasion, ulceration with submucosal undermining results in narrow mucosal *bridges* of tissue raised off the underlying submucosa but still attached at either end.

ULCERATIVE COLITIS AND PROCTITIS

Ulcerative colitis is a chronic inflammatory disease of unknown etiology, involving primarily the mucosa of the distal colon and rectum.[9] It usually affects patients in early adult life and is characterized by abdominal pain, diarrhea, and rectal bleeding. Diagnosis is made on the basis of characteristic abnormalities seen during sigmoidoscopy and on barium enema examinations.[9,14,30] Since infectious colitis may simulate ulcerative colitis, intestinal infections must be excluded.[27]

The sigmoidoscopic findings in the mildest form of ulcerative colitis are edema and erythema.[14,30] As the disease becomes more advanced, granularity and friability first appear and then become more prominent (Fig. 11-4). In severe ulcerative colitis, friability is spontaneous and most of the inflamed mucosa is covered with fresh blood (Fig. 11-5). The rectal valves become blunted and the rectosigmoid colon may not be distensible with air insufflation. Since the disease involves the mucosa in a diffuse and superficial pattern, discrete ulceration is seldom seen. The lumen often contains copious amounts of exudate that adheres to the wall of the rectum and colon. In advanced and chronic disease, pseudopolyp formation may occur and strictures may develop. There is nearly universal involvement of the rectum in ulcerative colitis and the inflammatory process often becomes less evident proximally. Most of the abnormalities described above are nonspecific and may, on occasion, be present in other forms of colitis, such as infectious colitis or Crohn's colitis. Flexible sigmoidoscopy can be safely performed in patients with active ulcerative colitis, but air insufflation should be kept to a minimum and advancement of the endoscope tip performed gently and only under direct visualization. It is usually only necessary to visualize the rectum in order to make a visual diagnosis and obtain mucosal biopsies.

Ulcerative proctitis is a variant of ulcerative colitis limited to the rectum. The characteristic clinical features are frequent passage of blood and mucus, tenesmus, and only minor alterations in bowel habits. Mucosal abnormalities are similar to those described above for ulcerative colitis. The pathognomonic finding that suggest the diagnosis of ulcerative proctitis is the sharp cut-off between the proctitis and proximal normal rectum or lower sigmoid colon (Fig. 11-6). This sharp demarcation occurs anywhere from 5 to 15 cm from the anus.

CROHN'S DISEASE

Crohn's disease is a chronic inflammatory disease of the gastrointestinal tract that may involve any segment of the gut but most commonly involves the distal ileum and right colon.[10] The inflammatory
process is transmural and also affects the adjacent mesentery and lymph
nodes. The clinical course is prolonged and variable and often complicated by perianal disease with fissures and fistulae. The disease process
is often discontinuous, with skip areas of involvement throughout the
bowel.

The sigmoidoscopic appearance of Crohn's disease, when the rectum is involved, is usually different from that seen in ulcerative colitis,
although on occasion the gross appearance may closely resemble that
of ulcerative colitis. Approximately half of patients with Crohn's disease
have no involvement of the rectosigmoid mucosa or only mild edema
and erythema secondary to chronic diarrhea. Rectal biopsies of normal
or only minimally abnormal mucosa may on occasion show histologic
presence of the granulomas that are characteristic of Crohn's disease.
When the rectum is involved, it may show evidence of cobblestoning
as the characteristic morphologic feature. This cobblestone appearance
usually results from islands of mucosa separated by linear ulcerations.
Normal rectal vasculature is usually obscured by edema and erythema.
Discrete ulcerations are more frequently seen in Crohn's disease than
in ulcerative colitis and often occur in areas of relatively normal mucosa.
The ulcerations are variable and may be rounded, serpiginous, or linear
(Fig. 11-7) and are often quite deep (Fig. 11-8). Pseudopolyps also occur
in Crohn's disease and do not distinguish this disease from ulcerative
colitis. Undermining submucosal ulcers may result in *mucosal bridging*,
which may be impressive on occasion (Fig. 11-9). In order to obtain
histologic confirmation, biopsies should be obtained from the edge of
ulcerations as well as from diffusely inflamed and even normal appearing mucosa.

ANTIBIOTIC-ASSOCIATED (PSEUDOMEMBRANOUS) COLITIS

Pseudomembranous enterocolitis was previously a rare entity
reported in the setting of uremia, shock, sepsis, or colonic obstruction.
Most cases now are seen in association with antibiotic usage.[4,28] The
etiology of this process appears to be a toxin or toxins produced by the
organism *Clostridium difficile*. Antibiotic-associated colitis is usually
diagnosed by sigmoidoscopy with or without biopsy and/or demonstrating the presence of *C. difficile* toxin in the stool.

The changes noted during flexible sigmoidoscopy are raised yellow-ish-white plaque-like lesions that vary in size from a few mm to 1–2 cm (Fig. 11-10). In rare advanced cases an entire pseudomembrane may line the colon. The intervening mucosa between these plaques is normal or shows nonspecific edema and erythema. The sigmoid colon and rectum is involved in the majority of patients; however, the process may be limited to the more proximal or even the right colon in some circumstances.[7,26] One recent study found that 60-cm flexible sigmoidoscopy would detect mucosal abnormalities in 91% of patients with the disease.[26]

ISCHEMIC COLITIS

Ischemic colitis results from inadequate tissue perfusion secondary to occlusive or nonocclusive vascular disease leading to relative hypoxia of the colonic mucosa.[24] Ischemic colitis is variable in extent and severity ranging from mild nonspecific inflammatory changes of the mucosa to transmural necrosis with infarction. The areas of colon that are usually involved are the watershed areas between two adjacent arterial supplies (1) the splenic flexure of the colon between the superior and inferior mesenteric arteries, and (2) the rectosigmoid colon between the inferior mesenteric and internal iliac arteries. Most patients are elderly with evidence of generalized vascular disease and present with abdominal pain and rectal bleeding.

Findings during flexible sigmoidoscopy are variable and may be normal if the area of mucosa involved is above the level visualized. The range of mucosal abnormalities in ischemic colitis include nonspecific proctitis or colitis, discrete ulcers, nodular lesions, and an adherent membrane. A recent study defines three endoscopic stages (1) an acute stage characterized by petechiae, palor, and erythema; (2) a subacute stage consisting of ulceration and exudation (Fig. 11-11); and (3) a chronic stage characterized by stricture, decrease in haustrations, and mucosal granularity.[24] Mucosal biopsy may show findings suggesting ischemic necrosis but more often is nonspecific.

RADIATION COLITIS

Radiation therapy to a number of pelvic, intraabdominal, and retroperitoneal structures is complicated by radiation injury to the small bowel and colon in 5–15% of patients.[12,22] Damage usually occurs to both the small bowel and colon, and thus diagnosis of radiation-induced injury to one anatomic segment of gut (e.g., small bowel) should lead to the strong suspicion of damage to another segment as well (e.g., colon). The incidence of bowel injury is related to the total dose of radiation and usually becomes evident above 5000 rads. The pathologic changes have been divided into acute, subacute, and chronic phases.[22] The acute phase is characterized by edema, erythema, and inflammation of the mucosa. In the subacute phase, from 2 to 12 months after completion of radiotherapy, the submucosa becomes thickened and fibrotic. The chronic phase results from obliterative changes in the small arterioles leading to progressive ischemia. Ischemic ulceration may develop in the sigmoid colon or rectum, scarring with partial bowel obstruction may occur, and fistula formation with abscesses may erode into adjacent organs such as the vagina and bladder.

Sigmoidoscopy during the early acute phase demonstrates an edematous and slightly inflamed mucosa. Only with higher doses of radiotherapy is friability and ulceration noted. In the late phase, the mucosa becomes pale and opaque from submucosal fibrosis and edema. Prominent submucosal telangiectatic vessels may be noted in the more normal appearing mucosa (Fig. 11-12). Even in the chronic phase, active mucosal disease with erythema, friability, granularity, and overt ulceration may be seen. Rectosigmoid strictures are particularly common and may prevent advancement of the sigmoidoscope. The rectal strictures are usually located somewhat higher than the ulcerations, which are most often located on the anterior rectal wall 4–8 cm from the anus and are frequently transverse in orientation.

AMEBIC COLITIS

Amebiasis, which is caused by the organism *Entamoeba histolytica*, may be both an acute and chronic disease.[1] The colon is the usual site of initial disease and clinical manifestations vary from asymptomatic carriers to a severe fulminating colitis. The cecum is involved in the majority of chronic cases, and the rectum less often shows evidence of disease. Diagnosis rests on microbiologic study of stools and serologic tests, but sigmoidoscopy and biopsy may also be helpful in diagnosis.

Flexible sigmoidoscopy is valuable when the rectum or sigmoid colon is involved. Sigmoidoscopy should be performed without prior bowel preparation. The characteristic abnormality is discrete small ulcers covered by yellow-white exudate and bordered by raised and undermined edges.[1] In contrast to patients with ulcerative colitis and infectious colitis, the intervening mucosa is usually normal. However, exceptions to this characteristic picture may occur, and amebiasis may present with diffuse mucosal abnormalities and be mistaken for ulcerative colitis.[20] Biopsies are occasionally helpful if trophozoites can be identified.

DIVERTICULAR DISEASE

Diverticular disease of the colon is the term applied to both the presence of diverticulosis and its clinical consequences, diverticulitis and diverticular hemorrhage.[2,8] Diverticulosis represents herniation of the mucosa and submucosa through the muscular coat of the colonic wall to lie within the serosa and thus form a pseudodiverticulum. Diverticulitis is the inflammatory process that develops around a micro-perforation of the diverticulum. Diverticular hemorrhage most commonly originates from diverticula of the right colon and is not usually associated with pathologic evidence of diverticulitis. Asymptomatic diverticula are frequently visualized on the left side of the colon during 60-cm flexible sigmoidoscopy (Fig. 11-13). Diverticulitis with mild non-specific mucosal changes or luminal narrowing from surrounding inflammation, spasm, and fibrosis is seen less often.

The sigmoid colon is the most common site of diverticula and is involved in 95% of patients with diverticulosis. Diverticula may number from a few to several hundred and may have large diameters that simulate the colonic lumen. Great care with advancement of the sigmoidoscope tip should be taken to avoid entrance into a wide-mouthed diverticulum with resultant perforation by air insufflation or direct tip trauma.

Flexible sigmoidoscopy may be difficult in patients with diverticulitis. There is often marked sigmoid colon spasm and poor luminal distension that prevents advancement of the tip of the instrument. Diverticulitis may also be accompanied by fixed luminal narrowing by edema or scarring that will not allow further penetration of the instrument. In the area of diverticulitis, the colonic mucosa may show evidence of edema and erythema with focal petechial hemorrhage.

Bleeding from diverticulosis most often complicates diverticula of the right colon beyond the reach of the flexible sigmoidoscope. When diverticular bleeding occurs in the left colon, it is difficult to determine the actual bleeding diverticulum.

BENIGN AND MALIGNANT NEOPLASMS

Polypoid lesions of the rectosigmoid colon may be classified as (1) neoplastic polyps, both benign and malignant varieties; (2) nonneoplastic polyps, such as hyperplastic polyps and juvenile polyps; and (3) submucosal lesions, such as lipomas and leiomyomas.[5] Most patients with colonic polyps either are asymptomatic or have occult or overt rectal bleeding.

The most common neoplastic polyps are benign adenomatous polyps, which are classified histologically as tubular, tubulovillous, or pure villous adenomas. Adenomatous polyps may be either sessile (Figs. 11-14 and 11-15) or pedunculated (Fig. 11-16). The surface of the polyp is often irregular, erythematous, and friable and may contain clusters of tissue in a grape-like pattern. Epithelial dysplasia and invasive malignancy may occur focally within an adenomatous polyp. Biopsies of the polyp surface, therefore, are not adequate to exclude focal carcinoma, and total excision is needed for accurate histologic diagnosis.

Non-neoplastic polyps have a variable appearance. Hyperplastic polyps are usually small, averaging less than 0.5 cm, and most often sessile with mucosa similar to that of the surrounding colon (Fig. 11-17). Juvenile polyps are usually single, pedunculated, and larger in size ranging from 0.5–2 cm. The heads of these polyps are particularly erythematous and often very friable.

A number of lesions may develop in the submucosa and result in elevation of the overlying epithelium, producing a polypoid appearance. Biopsy of these polyps usually reveal normal colonic mucosa. Lipomas are particularly common submucosal lesions that may be identified by their soft malleable nature. These lesions are less often seen at flexible sigmoidoscopy since they tend to occur predominantly in the right colon, particularly in the area of the ileocecal valve (Fig. 11-18).

The inherited polyposis syndromes involving the colon include familial polyposis coli, Gardner's syndrome, and Turcot's syndrome.[5] In these patients, the colon is studded with innumerable polyps, usually over a hundred in number, that range in size from a few mm to several cm (Fig. 11-19).

Adenocarcinoma may occur in either the rectum or colon in two general morphologic forms: polypoid and annular.[31] The annular constricting type is most commonly seen in the distal colon. This variety of tumor is evident by the irregular mucosal changes with heaped-up erythematous and edematous mucosa that is ulcerated and friable. The polypoid lesion often has a central ulceration surrounded by irregular friable borders (Fig. 11-20) and may be large with partial obstruction of the lumen (Fig. 11-21). Multiple biopsies should be obtained from these lesions in order to confirm visual impressions of malignancy.

VASCULAR LESIONS OF THE COLON

A wide variety of vascular lesions may be found in the colon.[6] Arteriovenous malformations (vascular ectasias or angiodysplasias) are by far the most common vascular abnormality of the colon and together

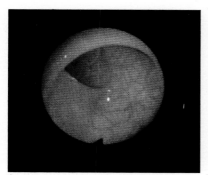

Figure 1. Normal colon. Pale pink mucosa and easily visible submucosal blood vessels.

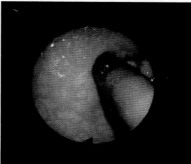

Figure 2. Normal distal rectum. Mucosa and instrument (black) seen during retroflexion of the flexible sigmoidoscope in the rectum.

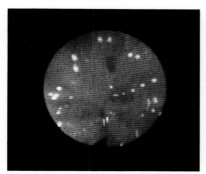

Figure 3. Internal hemorrhoids. Prominent veins and slightly inflamed mucosa evident during withdrawal of the sigmoidoscope through the anus.

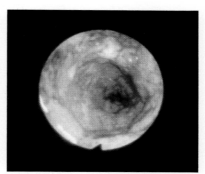

Figure 4. Ulcerative colitis. Mucosa of distal descending colon with spontaneous friability and moderate granularity.

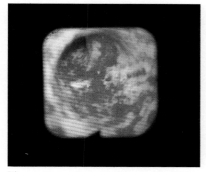

Figure 5. Severe ulcerative colitis. Spontaneous friability of the rectum with blood oozing from inflamed mucosa.

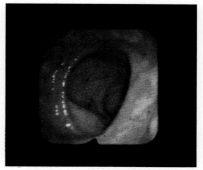

Figure 6. Ulcerative proctitis. Inflamed and ulcerated distal rectal mucosa (foreground) with sharp transition to normal mucosa above.

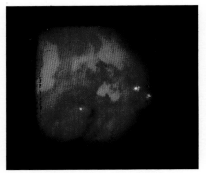

Figure 7. Crohn's colitis. Superficial ulcers of different shapes in edematous and erythematous rectal mucosa.

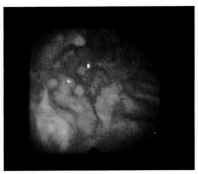

Figure 8. Crohn's colitis. Deep ulcers covered with white exudate.

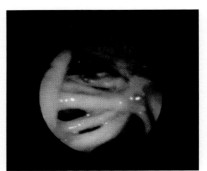

Figure 9. Mucosal bridging secondary to Crohn's colitis.

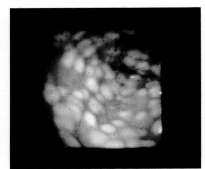

Figure 10. Antibiotic-associated (pseudomembranous) colitis. Numerous yellow-white, raised lesions in sigmoid colon.

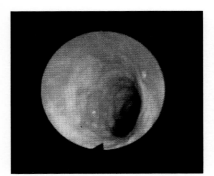

Figure 11. Ischemic colitis. Subacute stage of ischemic colitis with granularity, friability, exudate and large ulcers.

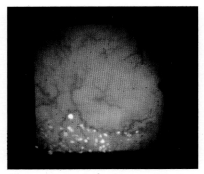

Figure 12. Radiation proctitis. Late stage with prominent submucosal telangiectatic vessels.

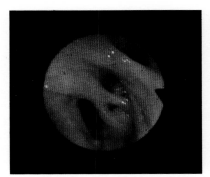

Figure 13. Diverticulosis. Numerous sigmoid colon diverticula with some simulating the colonic lumen.

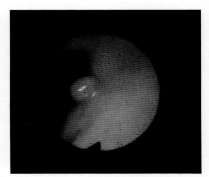

Figure 14. Small sessile polyps. Small round 0.5 cm adenomatous polyp in rectum.

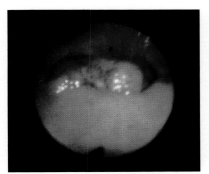

Figure 15. Large sessile polyps. Irregular sessile adenomatous polyp of rectum.

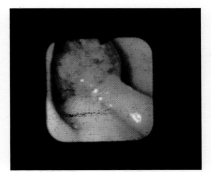

Figure 16. Pedunculated polyp. Benign adenomatous polyp with irregular, erythematous head and long stalk.

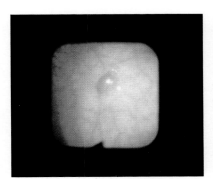

Figure 17. Hyperplastic polyp. Small 0.2 cm sessile polyp with mucosa identical to the surrounding colon.

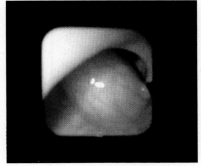

Figure 18. Lipoma. Submucosal smooth lesion of ileocecal valve with intact overlying mucosa.

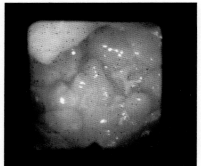

Figure 19. Polyposis coli. Multiple colonic polyps of variable sizes from patient with familial polyposis coli.

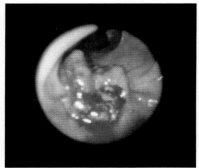

Figure 20. Adenocarcinoma, sigmoid colon. Flat tumor with irregular raised edges, central depression and spontaneous bleeding.

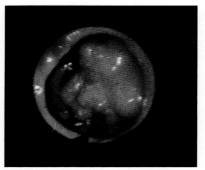

Figure 21. Obstructing polypoid adenocarcinoma. Large tumor partially obstructing distal descending colon.

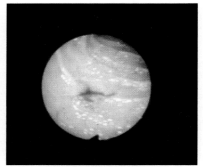

Figure 22. Arteriovenous malformation. Prominent telangiectatic lesion in colon.

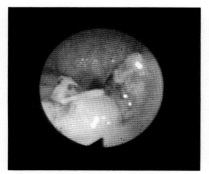

Figure 23. Colonic anastomosis. Lumen is narrowed by irregular mucosal folds with visible black suture material.

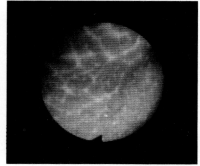

Figure 24. Melanosis coli. Brown-black discoloration of rectal mucosa.

with diverticular disease account for the majority of causes of massive lower gastrointestinal hemorrhage.[17] Arteriovenous malformations are associated with aging and found in patients over the age of 50–60 years. These lesions characteristically are multiple and usually occur in the cecum or ascending colon and thus require colonoscopy rather than sigmoidoscopy for diagnosis. Abdominal angiography is also utilized to make an accurate diagnosis. During colonoscopy for bleeding, visible prominent telangiectatic lesions associated with mucosal erosions have been identified most frequently (Fig. 11-22).

Hemangiomas are the second most common vascular lesion of the colon.[6] They most often occur as solitary lesions, but they may be multiple or occur as part of diffuse angiomatosis. Most hemangiomas are small and range from a few mm to 1–2 cm. Larger lesions, particularly in the rectum, have been identified in rare patients. Hemangiomas are raised, reddish-purple lesions that stand out from the mucosa. A distinct clinical form of hemangioma is the cavernous hemangioma of the rectum. These lesions are more extensive and often involve the entire rectum and some of the sigmoid colon. Diffuse vascular congestion and elevated nodules can be identified.

Colonic varices related to portal hypertension are very rare but may be a troublesome cause of rectal bleeding. These lesions are usually found in the rectosigmoid colon, and diagnosis is made by the presence of large venous structures projecting into the lumen of the colon.

Of the various hereditary vascular diseases, hereditary hemorrhagic telangiectasia (Osler-Weber-Rendu disease) is the most significant. The most characteristic symptom of this disease is recurrent epistaxis in childhood. These patients may also have telangiectasias on the lips, oral and nasal pharyngeal membranes, tongue, or hand. When the gastrointestinal tract is involved, telangiectasias are most common in the stomach and small bowel but are occasionally found in the colon. The lesions in the upper gastrointestinal tract are more likely to cause significant bleeding. At endoscopy the telangiectasias are bright, cherry-red lesions, 1–3 mm in diameter, and often appear similar to cutaneous spider angiomas seen in patients with cirrhosis.

SEXUALLY RELATED RECTOSIGMOID DISEASES

A wide variety of sexually transmitted intestinal diseases have been reported in homosexual men attending venereal disease clinics.[3,19,21] These diseases are probably related to a high carrier rate and the wide prevalence of oral–anal sexual activity. A large number of these intestinal infections have a predilection for the anus and rectum. Bacterial diseases that are commonly associated with proctitis include shigellosis, salmonellosis, campylobacteriosis, gonorrhea, syphilis, and chlamydial infection. Amebiasis is the only protozoan disease that is manifest by rectal ulceration. Viral disease more often involves the anus and includes herpes simplex and condyloma accuminatum. In addition, acquired immune deficiency syndrome (AIDS) and Kaposi's sarcoma may be virus-mediated diseases. Rigid sigmoidoscopy with disposable instruments is preferred by many clinics treating homosexual men with anorectal disease, because of concern regarding adequate disinfection of flexible sigmoidoscopes. Only a few of the venereal diseases of the rectum not reviewed in other parts of this chapter will be mentioned here.

In rectal gonorrhea, generalized erythema, edema, and a purulent exudate are most commonly seen. These mucosal findings are most prominent distally near the anorectal junction, and mucosal abnormalities only rarely extend beyond the rectum.

The usual finding in anorectal syphilis is a primary chancre on the skin around the anus. Rectal ulceration is occasionally observed during sigmoidoscopy, and rarely diffuse erythema and edema of the rectum has been reported. Syphilitic lesions may even resemble adenocarcinoma of the rectum on rare occasions.

Chlamydia ranks with the gonococcus as one of the most common sexually transmitted organisms. Bacteriologic and serologic testing is not sensitive or generally available, and thus a specific diagnosis is often not made. It is likely that much of the nonspecific proctitis in homosexual men is caused by *Chlamydia* of the non-LGV type. The usual picture with chlamydial infection is focal edema and erythema associated with friability in the rectum. Ulcerations are more commonly seen with LGV strains than with non-LGV organisms. In chronic LGV proctitis, by contrast, more severe proctocolitis and rectal strictures may develop.

Anorectal infection with herpes simplex virus may be both symptomatic and asymptomatic. The usual complaint is severe anorectal pain, rectal discharge, and constipation. Vesicles may be seen on the perianal skin and anal ulcerations may be evident. Sigmoidoscopy is often impossible or extremely difficult because of severe anal discomfort. If sigmoidoscopy is possible, erythema, edema, and some friability may be present in the rectum, but the sigmoid colon is not involved.

In Kaposi's sarcoma, purple nodular lesions similar to those seen on the skin may be seen in the colon. This tumor is often associated with acquired immune deficiency syndrome (AIDS) and may be present with a number of other infections.

Physicians evaluating homosexual men with anorectal symptoms should inquire regarding the use of foreign objects in the rectum. Anal and rectal mucosal inflammation due to trauma may be very difficult to differentiate from infectious agents. A clue to traumatic proctitis may be the presence of a nonspecific proctitis associated with anal fissures. A number of reports of actual laceration of the anterior rectosigmoid wall have been reported.

ABNORMALITIES OF THE POSTOPERATIVE COLON

Flexible sigmoidoscopy is performed on occasion to inspect colonic anastomoses following resection of tumors or Crohn's disease and also to inspect colostomies or ileostomies.

Colonic Anastomoses

Colonic anastomoses are usually readily evident during flexible sigmoidoscopy after resection of the rectum or sigmoid colon for adenocarcinoma, Crohn's disease, or other processes. Recurrent adenocarcinoma occasionally occurs at the site of anastomosis and needs to be distinguished from normal postoperative anastomotic mucosal changes. Normally a slight narrowing of the colonic lumen is evident at the site of the anastomosis, and suture material may be seen protruding into the lumen (Fig. 11-23). The mucosa at this junction may be slightly heaped-up and erythematous or even friable on occasion. Visual inspection is not reliable to distinguish a normal colonic anastomosis from recurrent carcinoma at the suture line, and thus multiple biopsies should be taken from the anastomosis, particularly in areas of erythema or friability.

Colostomies and Ileostomies

The flexible sigmoidoscope is occasionally used to examine colostomies and ileostomies for stomal dysfunction or to evaluate the proximal bowel. Digital examination of the stoma should be performed prior to endoscopy to determine the patency and size of the opening. Air insufflation can be difficult to maintain but should be employed to determine the direction of the lumen, since sharp right-angle turns are often present several centimeters below the anterior abdominal wall. The bowel is often sutured to the anterior abdominal wall and may be relatively fixed by adhesions in the postoperative state. In this situation, care should be taken to not forcibly insert the instrument when the lumen is not well visualized or the instrument is not sliding easily. Following total proctocolectomy, patients may have a standard ileostomy or a continent ileostomy (Kock pouch). Some of the patients with a Kock pouch have ileostomy dysfunction associated with inflammation of the mucosa consisting of erythema, friability, and erosions (pouchitis).[15]

MISCELLANEOUS RECTOSIGMOID FINDINGS

A few additonal entities that may be encountered during flexible sigmoidoscopy will be briefly mentioned.

Melanosis Coli

Melanosis coli is a benign and reversible condition found in some patients who use anthracene cathartics on a chronic basis (mean, 9 months).[11] There are also a few reports associating melanosis coli with carcinoma of the colon. The pigment, which resembles both melanin and lipofuscin, has not yet been identified. It most often is found in the cecum or rectum but may be distributed throughout the entire colon. The diagnosis of melanosis coli is usually made during sigmoidoscopy when a mucosal discoloration ranging from brown to black is noted (Fig. 11-24). Melanosis is usually darkest in the distal rectum and lighter in the higher rectum and sigmoid colon. Mucosal biopsy shows increased numbers of pigment-laden macrophages in the lamina propria.

Solitary Ulcer of the Rectum

Patients with the syndrome of solitary ulcer of the rectum usually present with alteration of their bowel habits, passage of blood, and mucus per rectum and anorectal pain.[13] In spite of the designation of this disease, not all patients have only a single ulcer. Approximately one-third of patients will have two or more ulcers in the rectum. Furthermore, a nodular or polypoid mucosa may be seen in addition to the rectal ulceration. Thus, patients with "solitary ulcer of the rectum" may have a single ulceration, multiple ulcerations, a discrete erythematous area of rectal mucosa, or a nodular and polypoid mucosa.

Pneumatosis Cystoides Intestinalis

Pneumatosis cystoides intestinalis is a rare gastrointestinal disease of unknown etiology that is characterized by the presence of gas-filled submucosal or subserosal cysts.[25] The sigmoidoscopic appearance of this entity consists of submucosal cystic lesions that project into the bowel lumen. The mucosa overlying the cyst is usually pale and transparent. These cysts are tense and firm and dramatically collapse when punctured.

Endometriosis

Endometriosis affects women in their middle and later reproductive years and may produce a wide variety of symptoms.[18] This disorder can involve both the colon and the small intestine. With rectosigmoid involvement, crampy abdominal pain, constipation, diarrhea, and tenesmus may be present. Luminal obstruction from this process may result in reduction in stool caliber and constipation. Hematochezia is a relatively uncommon occurrence. During flexible sigmoidoscopy, the most common abnormality is an obstructing extramucosal mass lesion and thus endoscopic biopsies are usually not diagnostic. Patients often exhibit extreme tenderness in the region of colonic endometriosis.

REFERENCES

1. Adams EB, MacLeod IN: Invasive amebiasis. I. Amebic dysentery and its complications. Medicine 56:315–323, 1977
2. Almy TP, Naitove A: Diverticular disease of the colon, in Sleisenger MH, Fordtran JS (Eds): Gastrointestinal Disease (3rd ed). Philadelphia, W.B. Saunders, 1983, pp 896–912
3. Baker RW, Peppercorn MA: Gastrointestinal ailments of homosexual men. Medicine 61:390–405, 1982
4. Bartlett JG: The pseudomembranous enterocolitides, in Sleisenger MH, Fordtran JS (Eds): Gastrointestinal Disease (3rd ed.). Philadelphia, W.B. Saunders, 1983, pp 1168–1184
5. Boland CR, Kim YS: Colonic polyps and the gastrointestinal polyposis syndromes, in Sleisenger MH, Fordtran JS (Eds): Gastrointestinal Disease (3rd ed.). Philadelphia, W.B. Saunders, 1983, pp 1196–1219
6. Boley SJ, Brandt LJ, Mitsudo SM: Vascular lesions of the colon. Adv Intern Med 29:301–326, 1984.
7. Burbige EJ, Radigan JJ: Antibiotic-associated colitis with normal-appearing rectum. Dis Colon Rectum 24:198–200, 1981
8. Cello JP: Diverticular disease of the colon. West J Med 134:515–523, 1981
9. Cello JP: Ulcerative colitis, in Sleisenger MH, Fordtran JS (Eds): Gastrointestinal Disease (3rd ed.). Philadelphia, W.B. Saunders, 1983, pp 1122–1168
10. Donaldson RM Jr: Crohn's disease, in Sleisenger MH, Fordtran JS (eds): Gastrointestinal Disease (3rd ed.). Philadelphia, W.B. Saunders, 1983, pp 1088–1121
11. Earnest DL: Other diseases of the colon and rectum, in Sleisenger MH, Fordtran JS (Eds): Gastrointestinal Disease (3rd ed.). Philadelphia, W.B. Saunders, 1983, pp 1294–1323.

12. Earnest DL, Trier JS: Radiation enteritis and colitis, in Sleisenger MH, Fordtran JS (Eds): Gastrointestinal Disease (3rd ed.). Philadelphia, W.B. Saunders, 1983, pp 1259–1268
13. Ford MJ, Anderson JR, Gilmour HM, et al.: Clinical spectrum of "solitary ulcer" of the rectum. Gastroenterology 84:1533–1540, 1983
14. Hogan WJ, Hensley GT, Geenen JE: Endoscopic evaluation of inflammatory bowel disease. Med Clin N Amer 64:1083–1102, 1980
15. Kelly DG, Phillips SF, Kelly KA, et al.: Dysfunction of the continent ileostomy: Clinical features and bacteriology. Gut 24:193–201, 1983
16. Kirsner JB: The irritable bowel syndrome: A clinical review and ethical considerations. Arch Intern Med 141:635–639, 1981
17. Meyer CT, Troncale FJ, Galloway S, Sheahan DG: Arteriovenous malformations of the bowel: An analysis of 22 cases and a review of the literature. Medicine 60:36–48, 1981
18. Meyers WC, Kelvin FM, Jones RS: Diagnosis and surgical treatment of colonic endometriosis. Arch Surg 114:169–175, 1979
19. Owen RL: Sexually related intestinal disease, in Sleisenger MH, Fordtran JS (Eds). Gastrointestinal Disease (3rd ed.). Philadelphia, W.B. Saunders, 1983, pp 966–985
20. Pittman FE, El-Hashimi WK, Pittman JC: Studies of human amebiasis. I. Clinical and laboratory findings in eight cases of acute amebic colitis. Gastroenterology 65:581–587, 1973
21. Quinn TC, Stamm WE, Goodell SE, et al.: The polymicrobial origin of intestinal infections in homosexual men. N Engl J Med 309:576–582, 1983
22. Reichelderfer M, Morrissey JF: Colonoscopy in radiation colitis. Gastrointest Endosc 26:41–43, 1980
23. Riddlesberger MM Jr, Lebenthal E: Nodular colonic mucosa of childhood: Normal or pathologic? Gastroenterology 79:265–270, 1980
24. Scowcroft CW, Sanowski RA, Kozarek RA: Colonoscopy in ischemic colitis. Gastrointest Endosc 27:156–161, 1981.
25. Shallal JA, van Heerden JA, Bartholomew LG, Cain JC: Pneumatosis cystoides intestinalis. Mayo Clin Proc 49:180–184, 1974
26. Tedesco FJ, Corless JK, Brownstein RE: Rectal sparing in antibiotic-associated pseudomembranous colitis: A prospective study. Gastroenterology 83:1259–1260, 1982.
27. Tedesco FJ, Hardin RD, Harper RN, Edwards BH: Infectious colitis endoscopically simulating inflammatory bowel disease: A prospective evaluation. Gastrointest Endosc 29:195–197, 1983.
28. Trnka YM, LaMont JT: Clostridium difficile colitis. Adv Intern Med 29:85–107, 1984.
29. Tucker H, Schuster MM: Irritable bowel syndrome: Newer pathophysiologic concepts. Adv Intern Med 27:183–204, 1982.
30. Waye JD: The role of colonoscopy in the differential diagnosis of inflammatory bowel disease. Gastrointest Endosc 23:150–154, 1977.
31. Winawer SJ, Sherlock P: Malignant neoplasms of the small and large intestine, in Sleisenger MH, Fordtran JS (Eds): Gastrointestinal Disease (3rd ed.). Philadelphia, W.B. Saunders, 1983, pp 1220–1249.

Index

t = table
fig = figure

153